If These Balls Could Talk

A Guide to Testicular Cancer

Testicular Cancer Foundation

ISBN Paperback: 978-1-969826-20-7
ISBN E-Book: 978-1-969826-21-4

First Edition

Published by Freiling Agency
Warrenton, VA
www.freilingagency.com

Foreword

When I was diagnosed with testicular cancer at 21 years old, I didn't know what I didn't know. I didn't know how common this cancer was. I didn't know how curable it is when caught early. And I definitely didn't know how many conversations were not happening because people were uncomfortable talking about bodies, symptoms, or fear.

That silence is dangerous.

If These Balls Could Talk exists to break it.

I'm excited about this book not because it's clever or provocative, though it is, but because it does something incredibly important. It makes education accessible. It meets people where they are. It takes a topic that is too often whispered about and brings it into the open in a way that is honest, human, and easy to understand.

Education saves lives. Full stop.

Testicular cancer is the most common cancer in young men, yet awareness is still shockingly low. Too many guys don't know how to check themselves. Too many don't feel comfortable asking questions. Too many diagnoses happen later than they should, not because the disease is sneaky, but because the conversation never started.

This book helps start that conversation.

Whether you're a patient, a survivor, a partner, a parent, a friend, or someone who just picked this up out of curiosity, my hope is that you walk away knowing more than you did before and feeling empowered to act on it. Knowledge reduces fear. Awareness creates confidence. And confidence leads to early detection.

That's why the Testicular Cancer Foundation exists. And that's why a book like this matters.

If this book prompts even one person to do a self exam, to see a doctor sooner, or to talk openly about testicular health without shame or hesitation, then it has done its job.

I'm proud of what this book represents. I'm proud of the education it delivers. And I'm excited about the lives it has the potential to impact.

Let's keep talking.

Matt Ferstler
Founder, Testicular Cancer Foundation

Contents

IF THESE BALLS COULD TALK

Chapter 1

What is Testicular Cancer?

Testicular Cancer is the most common cancer in men aged 15-35. Even though it's not the most common cancer overall, it packs a punch for those it affects. This chapter breaks down what testicular cancer is, the different types, and how it impacts your body and mind.

Defining Testicular Cancer

Here's the deal: testicular cancer happens when rogue cells start growing uncontrollably in one or both of your testicles. The testicles, or testes, are a crucial part of the male reproductive system, producing sperm and testosterone—the hormone responsible for male development and reproduction. They sit inside the scrotum, that skin pouch below the penis.

Cancer starts when the normal cells in the testicle change and go out of control, dividing uncontrollably and forming a tumor. No one has pinpointed exactly why it happens. Still, most experts believe it's a combination of genetic, environmental, and lifestyle factors that contribute to the issue, similar to all other cancers.

Types of Testicular Cancer

Testicular cancer isn't just one kind of disease; it's a group of different types, each with its own traits, treatment options, and outlook. Knowing these types matters because the kind of testicular cancer you're dealing with can seriously impact your treatment path and what you can expect down the line.

1. Germ Cell Tumors

Germ cell tumors (GCTs) are the most common type of testicular cancer, making up over 90% of cases. Germ cells are the sperm producers, so it makes sense that most cancers in the testicles start here. Germ cell tumors break down into two main subtypes:

Seminomas are slow-growing cancers that are typically less aggressive than other types of cancer. They generally respond well to treatment and are often detected early because they tend to cause noticeable symptoms. Seminomas usually occur in men aged 25 to 45 and make up about half of all testicular cancer cases. They are further classified into two types:

Classical Seminomas: These are the most common type of seminoma, usually diagnosed in men in their 30s and 40s.

Spermatocytic Seminomas: Although rarer, spermatocytic seminomas usually occur in older men (typically over 50) and are often even less aggressive.

Non-Seminomas: Non-seminomas are generally faster-growing and more aggressive than seminomas. They often affect younger men (usually in their teens to early 30s) and require more intensive treatment. Non-seminomas can consist of one or a combination of four distinct cell types:

Embryonal Carcinoma: A fast-growing type that can spread quickly to other parts of the body.

Yolk Sac Carcinoma: The most common type of testicular cancer in children, but it also occurs in adults.

Choriocarcinoma: A rare and aggressive form of testicular cancer that can spread quickly.

Teratoma: Made up of various types of tissue, teratomas can grow aggressively and spread, but they generally do not spread as fast as other non-seminomas.

2. Stromal Tumors

Stromal tumors account for only about 5% of adult testicular cancers but are more common in young boys. They develop in the supportive and hormone-producing tissues of the testicles rather than the germ cells. Two primary types of stromal tumors are:

Leydig Cell Tumors: These tumors arise from Leydig cells, which produce testosterone. Although usually benign, they can sometimes be malignant and spread to other areas of the body.

Sertoli Cell Tumors: Arising from Sertoli cells that support and nourish sperm cells, these tumors are typically benign but can occasionally be malignant.

3. Secondary Testicular Cancer

Secondary testicular cancer is when cancer from another part of the body spreads (metastasizes) to the testicles. This type is rare and typically occurs with cancers of the lymphatic system (like lymphoma) or prostate cancer. Treatment for secondary testicular cancer is usually based on the origin of the primary cancer rather than typical testicular cancer treatments.

Overview of the Disease and Its Impact

Testicular cancer might be relatively rare, with around 9,500 new cases in the U.S. each year, but it hits hard—especially since it often strikes men right in their prime. Most guys dealing with this are young, active, and just starting to build their careers, relationships, and families. Getting a cancer diagnosis at this stage in life can rock you emotionally, physically, and socially.

1. Physical Impact

Symptoms of testicular cancer often include a painless lump or swelling in the testicle, a feeling of heaviness in the scrotum, and sometimes pain or discomfort. Not every lump means cancer, but any change needs to be checked right away to rule out serious issues.

When caught early, testicular cancer has one of the highest survival rates out there. With treatments like surgery, chemo, and radiation, most guys diagnosed at an early stage can expect a full recovery. But let's be real—the treatments can come with their own set of side effects, hitting both short-term and long-term health, including potential fertility issues, hormone imbalances, and changes in sexual function.

2. Impact on Fertility and Sexual Health

For a lot of men, a big concern with testicular cancer is how it's going to affect their fertility and sexual health. The testicles are central to producing both sperm and testosterone, so treatment can hit these functions hard. The most common initial treatment is surgery to remove a testicle (orchiectomy), which can lower testosterone levels if only one testicle is left. Chemo and radiation can also reduce sperm production, sometimes temporarily and sometimes permanently, so fertility preservation is a major consideration.

Guys facing these issues should talk about options like sperm banking before starting treatment and hormone replacement therapy if testosterone levels take a hit. Gaining a better understanding of these effects can significantly improve the quality of life for survivors. It is worth mentioning that although TC can impact testosterone and fertility, it isn't always the case!

3. Emotional and Psychological Impact

Getting diagnosed with testicular cancer can hit you like a freight train. Young men often feel completely blindsided, trying to cope with a complex mix of emotions—fear, anger, confusion, and sadness. The physical changes from surgery or treatment can stir up concerns about body image, identity, and masculinity. Sometimes, these emotional punches can be just as tough as the physical ones.

For a lot of guys, talking to a therapist or joining a support group, like those offered by the Testicular Cancer Foundation, can make a real difference. Having a solid support network helps men process what they're going through, cuts down on the feeling of isolation, and connects them with others who get it.

4. Social and Economic Impact

Testicular cancer can throw your whole life off track, messing with your relationships, work, and finances. Treatment often means taking time off work, which can be challenging if you have a demanding job or don't have flexible benefits. Medical bills pile up fast—even with insurance—and the recovery time can take a toll on your income and career progress.

On top of that, relationships get tested as partners, family, and friends try to step up and support you. Open communication and understanding in these relationships are crucial to getting through the changes that cancer brings.

Looking Ahead

Testicular cancer is serious, no doubt, but it's also highly treatable, especially if you catch it early. Education and awareness make all the difference—they're the keys to helping men understand the risks, recognize the symptoms, and get help when it's needed. Regular self-exams, getting checked out for anything unusual, and being willing to talk openly about men's health can truly save lives.

In the chapters ahead, we'll dig into every aspect of testicular cancer, from understanding the stages of the disease to exploring treatment options and survivorship. As you go through this book, keep in mind that knowledge is power. Whether you're here for yourself or to support someone else, understanding testicular cancer is a big step toward facing this with strength, purpose, and hope.

Chapter 2

Early Signs and Diagnosis

One of the tough things about testicular cancer is that it usually doesn't cause any pain or discomfort in the early stages, so a lot of guys end up overlooking the signs or putting off getting checked. Here are some key signs that all young men need to keep an eye out for:

Lump or Swelling in the Testicle

A lump or swelling in one testicle is one of the most common early signs of testicular cancer. This lump is usually painless, which can contribute to delays in diagnosis. Any noticeable change in the size, shape, or texture of the testicles should be examined by a healthcare provider as soon as possible.

Feeling of Heaviness or Dull Ache in the Lower Abdomen or Scrotum

Some men report a feeling of heaviness or a persistent dull ache in the lower abdomen, scrotum, or groin area. Although this symptom can be attributed to other conditions, it's important to get it checked if it doesn't go away.

Pain or Discomfort in a Testicle or the Scrotum

While testicular cancer is often painless, some men may experience intermittent or continuous discomfort in one testicle or the scrotum. Pain, even if mild, should be evaluated by a healthcare provider.

Changes in the Feel of the Testicle

Changes in texture, such as hardness or a rough or irregular surface, can also be warning signs. It's essential to be aware of any differences between the two testicles and to seek medical advice if anything feels unusual.

Unexpected Fluid Collection in the Scrotum

Known as a hydrocele, a sudden accumulation of fluid in the scrotum can be another early sign. This fluid buildup can cause swelling and discomfort.

Breast Growth or Soreness

Certain types of testicular cancer produce hormones that can cause breast tissue growth or soreness. While this symptom is less common, it's worth noting any unexpected changes in the chest area.

Persistent Back Pain

Although back pain can have many causes, persistent pain in the back, especially if coupled with other symptoms, can sometimes be associated with testicular cancer that has spread to lymph nodes in the lower back.

Being aware of these symptoms is crucial for catching testicular cancer early. Knowing what to watch for and performing regular self-exams can help you spot any unusual changes and consult a doctor before the issue becomes serious.

Diagnostic Methods for Testicular Cancer

If you or someone you know notices any of the signs listed above, the next step is to undergo diagnostic testing. Here are some commonly used methods to diagnose testicular cancer:

Self-Examination

Regular self-examinations are a crucial preventive measure for detecting testicular cancer early. Performing a self-exam monthly allows men to become familiar with the size, shape, and texture of their testicles, making it easier to notice any abnormalities. It's recommended to do the self-exam in the shower when the scrotum is relaxed. Any lumps, changes in size or shape, or areas of tenderness should be noted and brought to a doctor's attention.

Ultrasound

An ultrasound is typically the first test performed if a lump is detected in the testicle. This non-invasive imaging technique uses high-frequency sound waves to create images of the testicle's interior, helping to determine whether the lump is solid (which may indicate cancer) or filled with fluid (which is usually benign). An ultrasound can also reveal other characteristics that can help distinguish between benign and malignant growths.

Blood Tests

Some types of testicular cancer release specific proteins known as tumor markers into the bloodstream. A blood test can detect elevated levels of these markers, which include alpha-fetoprotein (AFP), human chorionic gonadotropin (HCG), and lactate dehydrogenase (LDH). While not all testicular tumors produce these markers, their presence can be an important indicator in diagnosing and tracking the progress of treatment. Elevated tumor markers can also aid in determining the type of testicular cancer.

Physical Examination

A thorough physical exam by a healthcare provider is an essential component of diagnosing testicular cancer. During the exam, the doctor will assess both testicles for any lumps, swelling, or changes in size and consistency. This exam is also an opportunity for the doctor to discuss symptoms and medical history to understand potential risk factors.

Biopsy (Rarely Used)

Unlike other cancers, a biopsy is not typically performed if testicular cancer is suspected due to the risk of spreading the cancer. Instead, if a testicular tumor is strongly suspected, doctors may recommend an orchiectomy, which is the surgical removal of the affected testicle. The tissue is then examined to confirm the diagnosis. Biopsies are generally only performed if the testicle is removed, allowing the medical team to confirm the presence and type of cancer cells without risking spread.

Imaging Tests

If testicular cancer is suspected or has been confirmed, additional imaging tests such as a CT scan or MRI may be used to check for cancer spread (metastasis). These scans help determine if the cancer has spread to lymph nodes, the lungs, or other parts of the body. Knowing the extent of the cancer's spread is essential for staging the disease and planning the most effective treatment.

Importance of Early Detection

Catching testicular cancer early can make a huge difference in treatment outcomes. Stats show a 99% five-year survival rate for cases where the cancer hasn't spread beyond the testicle. Even if it spreads to nearby lymph nodes or organs, there are solid treatments that lead to high survival rates.

Finding it early often means simpler, less aggressive treatments that keep side effects down and quality of life up. Men who know the signs and do regular self-exams can spot changes early, giving themselves the best shot at a full recovery.

Active Awareness

Knowing the signs of testicular cancer and using today's diagnostic tools can lead to early detection and better survival rates. Young men need to take charge of their health by learning how to do self-exams and recognizing the early warning signs of testicular cancer. By staying informed and proactive, men can catch changes early, get medical advice fast, and increase their chances of beating this disease.

Remember, knowing your body and paying attention to even small changes can make a big difference. Testicular cancer might be rare, but it's serious and requires vigilance. By discussing it, sharing our knowledge, and supporting one another in taking preventive steps, we can help protect young men and potentially save lives.

Chris' Story: From Fear to Gratitude

In 2016, at the age of 32, Chris from Germany received news that would change his life forever: a diagnosis of testicular cancer. At the time, his wife was pregnant with their second daughter, and what should have been a season of joyful anticipation quickly became a period of uncertainty and fear.

"I was diagnosed early, thankfully, and avoided chemotherapy and radiation. After surgery to remove the 'bad boy,' the plan was to monitor every three months," Chris recalls. But there was a moment in the hospital that shook him to his core. "My thyroid levels were too high for the CT scan contrast agent, so they couldn't confirm if the cancer had spread. That night, lying in the hospital, I woke up terrified—will I even live to see my daughter's birth?"

That sleepless night became a turning point. Chris emerged from the fear with a new perspective. "There's a before and an after," he says. "What seemed important—like the latest iPhone—just doesn't matter anymore. Now, it's the small things: my kids' smiles and family time. Those are the treasures."

While Chris avoided the physical toll of chemo or radiation, the emotional weight was heavy. "I wish I had been offered counseling, especially in the beginning. Support from a group like TCF made all the difference—it connected me with brothers who truly understood."

IF THESE BALLS COULD TALK

Chapter 3

The Stages of Testicular Cancer

Knowing the stages of testicular cancer is crucial for making smart treatment decisions and understanding what to expect. Staging is a way to describe how far the cancer has spread, and for testicular cancer, it usually follows the TNM system—Tumor, Node, and Metastasis. This chapter breaks down each stage, covering what it means, how it shapes treatment options, and what the outlook is for each level.

What is Testicular Cancer?

Testicular cancer kicks off when abnormal cells in the testicles start growing out of control. The testicles, sitting in the scrotum, are in charge of producing sperm and testosterone—the hormone that's key to male reproductive health. While it's rare, testicular cancer is still the most common cancer in young men aged 15 to 35.

The Importance of Staging in Testicular Cancer

Staging testicular cancer is a critical process in cancer diagnosis and treatment planning. Staging helps determine the extent of the cancer, guiding the medical team in recommending the most effective treatments. Diagnostic tests, such as imaging scans and blood tests, assess the size of the tumor and whether it has spread, forming the basis for staging.

Seek Treatment at High-Volume Centers

Where you receive treatment matters as much as the treatment itself, high-volume testicular cancer centers—those that treat a significant number of cases annually—consistently demonstrate better patient outcomes. These specialized centers have surgeons and oncologists with extensive experience in the nuances of testicular cancer staging, surgical techniques, and treatment protocols. Their multidisciplinary teams stay current with the latest research and have encountered the full spectrum of presentations, from straightforward cases to complex scenarios. Studies show that patients treated at high-volume centers experience fewer complications, more accurate staging, better preservation of fertility when possible, and improved long-term survival rates. If you've been diagnosed, it's worth traveling to reach a center with proven expertise in testicular cancer. Your life may depend on that decision. But here is how the cancer is staged:

Testicular cancer is generally staged using the TNM system, focusing on three key aspects:

Tumor (T): Refers to the size and extent of the primary tumor within the testicle.

Node (N): Indicates whether the cancer has spread to nearby lymph nodes.

Metastasis (M): Describes whether the cancer has spread to distant organs or tissues.

Stages of Testicular Cancer

The stages of testicular cancer range from 0 to 3, with each stage representing a different level of progression.

Stage 0: Carcinoma in Situ (CIS)

Description: Stage 0, also known as carcinoma in situ (CIS), indicates that abnormal cells are present in the lining of the seminiferous tubules, the structures within the testicle where sperm are produced. However, these cells haven't spread beyond this layer.

Implications: Carcinoma in situ is considered a precancerous condition rather than a full-blown cancer. Although CIS does not yet invade other tissues, it has the potential to develop into invasive cancer if left untreated. Treatment options for CIS may include careful monitoring (surveillance) or surgical removal of the affected tissue to prevent progression.

Stage 1: Localized Cancer

Stage 1A

Description: Cancer is confined to the testicle and has not spread to nearby lymph nodes or other parts of the body. The tumor remains limited to the testicle and the epididymis without signs of invasion into blood vessels or lymphatic vessels.

Implications: Stage 1A testicular cancer has an excellent prognosis, with a high cure rate. Treatment often involves a surgery called orchiectomy to remove the affected testicle. After surgery, patients may be placed under surveillance or given additional treatments based on individual circumstances.

Stage 1B

Description: The cancer is still confined to the testicle but has invaded blood vessels or lymphatic vessels within the testicle. This slight spread within the testicle distinguishes it from Stage 1A.

Implications: Like Stage 1A, the prognosis for Stage 1B remains highly favorable. Treatment typically includes orchiectomy, followed by either surveillance or additional treatments such as radiation or chemotherapy, depending on the risk factors.

Stage 2: Regional Spread

Now we're moving into Stage 2, where the cancer has spread beyond the testicle and into the lymph nodes in the abdomen. This is what we call "regional spread." At this stage, the cancer hasn't hit distant organs yet, but it's reaching out, so the treatment approach needs to be a bit more aggressive. Here's a breakdown of the levels within Stage 2:

Stage 2A

Description: Cancer has reached nearby lymph nodes in the abdomen, but these lymph nodes are still pretty small (less than 2 centimeters in size).

Implications: For Stage 2A, treatment may involve surgery to remove the affected lymph nodes (called retroperitoneal lymph node dissection) or chemotherapy to knock out any remaining cancer cells. The prognosis is still solid with proper treatment, but things are getting a little more intense.

Stage 2B

Description: Cancer has spread to abdominal lymph nodes that are now between 2 and 5 centimeters.

Implications: Treatment at this level usually includes a combination of surgery and chemotherapy. While the outlook remains positive, treatment becomes more intensive to make sure nothing is left behind.

Stage 2C

Description: Cancer has reached lymph nodes in the abdomen, and the affected lymph nodes are larger than 5 centimeters.

Implications: For Stage 2C, treatment ramps up. Surgery combined with a solid round of chemotherapy is the usual plan. The prognosis is still good, but patients will need close follow-ups and check-ins to make sure the cancer stays down.

Stage 3: Distant Spread

When we're talking Stage 3, cancer has spread beyond the regional lymph nodes. This is where it begins to spread to distant lymph nodes or organs, such as the lungs, or even farther, in rare cases, to organs like the liver or brain. At this stage, the cancer is more aggressive, but with modern treatment options, the outlook can still be strong. Let's break down the sub-stages within Stage 3:

Stage 3A

Description: Cancer has spread to distant lymph nodes or the lungs, with only slightly elevated levels of tumor markers (like AFP, HCG, and LDH) in the blood.

Implications: Treatment typically involves chemotherapy as the primary approach, aiming to hit all cancer cells throughout the body. The prognosis is still positive, but the treatment plan is more rigorous.

Stage 3B

Description: Cancer has spread to distant lymph nodes, the lungs, or possibly other organs, with moderate elevation in tumor markers.

Implications: Stage 3B requires an aggressive treatment approach, with chemotherapy as the main tool, sometimes combined with surgery to clear out remaining cancer cells. The prognosis remains hopeful, but it depends on how the body responds to therapy.

Stage 3C

Description: This is the most advanced stage. Cancer has spread to distant organs, which may include the lungs, liver, or brain, and tumor marker levels are significantly elevated.

Implications: Stage 3C is treated with intensive chemotherapy, and in some cases, surgery or radiation may be necessary to control the disease. The prognosis varies here depending on how far the cancer has spread and how well it responds to treatment. It's a tough battle, but one that modern medicine has made very successful for many men.

Prognosis and Treatment Overview

When it comes to testicular cancer, understanding the stage is key to knowing what lies ahead. The good news is that even in the advanced stages, treatments are often successful, and the survival rates are high compared to many other cancers. Here's a quick look at what the journey looks like at different stages:

Stage 0 to Stage 1: For men in these stages, treatment usually involves surgery to remove the affected testicle (orchiectomy). The five-year survival rate is incredibly high—almost 100%. After surgery, men are often placed under surveillance or given follow-up treatment like radiation or chemotherapy if the risk factors call for it. Most men in these early stages bounce back with full recoveries.

Stage 2: This is where surgery often combines with chemotherapy to make sure any spreading cancer cells are taken out. The survival rates are still very high, and the majority of men in this stage recover fully, though the treatment process may be a little tougher and require more follow-up care.

Stage 3: Now we're in advanced territory. Treatment will be a combination of chemotherapy, surgery, and sometimes radiation, especially if the cancer has spread to organs like the lungs. It's a tougher road, but with modern treatments, many men still come through with positive outcomes. Survival rates stay strong, though every case is unique.

The bottom line is that testicular cancer is a serious diagnosis, but it's also one with a strong chance of survival, especially if it's caught early. No matter the stage, having a solid understanding of what you're dealing with and knowing your options is crucial.

What to Expect and How to Prepare

Going through a cancer diagnosis and treatment can feel like a major disruption to life, but the more you know, the better prepared you'll be. Here are a few things to keep in mind:

Get Educated: Understand the stage and type of cancer you have. Knowing the details helps you feel more in control and makes it easier to discuss your options with your medical team.

Build a Support Network: Don't go through this alone. Lean on family, friends, and support groups. Organizations like the Testicular Cancer Foundation offer resources and survivor networks where guys can connect with others who've been there.

Take Care of Yourself: Treatment can be physically and mentally demanding. Stay as physically active as you can, eat well, and keep a positive mindset. Mental toughness goes a long way in pushing through the rough patches.

Ask Questions: Never hesitate to ask your doctor about anything you don't understand. This is your health, your life—make sure you know what's going on every step of the way.

Stay on Top of Follow-Up Care: After treatment, you'll need regular check-ups to make sure everything stays clear. Stick to the schedule, get those scans, and keep your doctor in the loop with any changes.

Treatment Preparation

Understanding the stages of testicular cancer isn't just about learning medical terms—it's about knowing exactly what you're up against and taking control of your fight. The more you know, the better you can plan and the stronger you'll feel. This isn't an easy road, but you're not the first to walk it. With the right knowledge, a solid plan, and a strong support network, you're ready to take on whatever comes next.

IF THESE BALLS COULD TALK

Chapter 4

Risk Factors and Prevention

When it comes to testicular cancer, knowing the risk factors and making smart choices can put you in a better position to stay ahead. Testicular cancer might not have a single clear cause, but there are a few risk factors that can increase the odds. This chapter lays out what you need to know about the genetic and environmental factors, lifestyle adjustments that could help, and the impact of alcohol and tobacco.

Genetic and Environmental Risk Factors

Testicular cancer doesn't care who you are or how strong you feel, but some risk factors make it more likely. Knowing what they are can make a difference.

Family History If cancer runs in your family, particularly if a father or brother has had testicular cancer, your chances are higher. Genetics plays a role, and while it doesn't guarantee you'll get cancer, it does mean you should be more vigilant. Keeping track of any changes and doing regular self-exams becomes even more important if testicular cancer is in your family tree.

Age and Race This cancer usually hits men between 15 and 35, right when most guys are building their lives. Testicular cancer is also more common in white men than in other racial groups. No one's exactly sure why, but the pattern is there. If you're a young man, especially a white one, keep an eye on things.

Undescended Testicle (Cryptorchidism) If you were born with one or both testicles not fully descended (a condition known as cryptorchidism), you've got a higher risk. Even if surgery corrected it, men who had undescended testicles are more likely to face testicular cancer down the road. This makes regular self-checks and check-ups even more crucial.

Personal History of Testicular Cancer If you've had testicular cancer in one testicle, there's a slightly higher chance it could happen in the other. After beating cancer once, it might be easy to think you're done with it. But if you've been down this road, staying on top of self-exams and follow-up visits is essential to catching any recurrence early.

HIV/AIDS Men with HIV, especially those with AIDS, face a higher risk of developing testicular cancer. HIV weakens the immune system, which can impact the body's ability to fend off abnormal cell growth. If you're managing this condition, have regular screenings and talk to your doctor about extra precautions.

Lifestyle Adjustments to Reduce Risk

Some risk factors are out of your hands, but there's a lot you can do to keep yourself in top shape and potentially reduce the risk.

Self-Exams One of the most effective things you can do is to know your body through regular self-exams. Doing a quick self-check once a month helps you get familiar with the usual size, shape, and feel of your testicles. If something changes—a lump, a bump, or a new tenderness—you'll notice it quickly. This simple habit, done in the shower or whenever you're relaxed, can be the difference between early detection and a tougher fight.

Exercise and Diet Staying active and eating right doesn't directly prevent testicular cancer, but it strengthens your body. When your body's in top form, your immune system and recovery potential are both improved. Exercise also helps with circulation and stress management, both of which play a role in keeping you resilient. So keep moving, whether it's lifting weights, running, or playing sports—just stay active.

Avoiding Harmful Chemicals There's some evidence that exposure to certain chemicals, like pesticides or industrial solvents, might increase cancer risk. If you work with these, make sure you're using proper protective gear and following safety protocols. It might seem excessive, but reducing exposure to potential carcinogens is worth the precaution. The risks may seem small now, but over a lifetime, exposure adds up.

Stress Management Let's get one thing straight—managing stress isn't about being soft. Chronic stress affects your immune system, making you more vulnerable to all kinds of health issues.

Find something that helps you release that tension, whether it's lifting, running, boxing, or a hobby that helps you unwind. Strong mental health keeps your body running smoothly and ready to handle challenges.

The Influence of Alcohol and Tobacco

These might not be the main causes of testicular cancer, but they do impact your overall health in ways that make it harder to fight off disease. Here's what to keep in mind about alcohol and tobacco use.

Alcohol While there's no direct link between moderate drinking and testicular cancer, heavy drinking does mess with your body's defenses. Alcohol weakens your immune system, stresses your liver, and impacts overall cellular health. It's not about going dry—just keep it moderate. Heavy drinking piles on health risks that could complicate things if you ever do face cancer.

Tobacco Now, tobacco's a different story. Smoking has a direct link to many cancers, and while the link to testicular cancer is still being researched, it's not worth the gamble. Cigarettes contain chemicals that harm your DNA and weaken your body's defenses over time. Quitting isn't easy, but the long-term benefits are huge—not just for avoiding cancer but for heart and lung health, too. Chewing tobacco isn't much better; the risks are still there.

Taking Control

You can't change your genetics or your race, but you can control a lot when it comes to lifestyle choices. Here's a straightforward game plan:

Know Your Body Get in the habit of doing monthly self-exams. You know your body better than anyone, so it makes sense to stay tuned into any changes. If something feels off, it's better to get it checked early.

Stay Active Regular exercise keeps you in fighting shape. A strong body is a resilient one, and that matters if you ever have to face down a diagnosis. Keeping your body moving builds strength, endurance, and overall health, which are essential assets in any health battle.

Limit Alcohol and Quit Tobacco Enjoying life is one thing, but moderation is key. Cutting down on alcohol and ditching tobacco are two of the most effective things you can do to strengthen your body's defenses. It's one less battle for your body to fight.

Routine Check-Ups Even if you're feeling fine, regular check-ups are smart. Routine visits help catch any changes early. If you've got any family history or previous conditions, keeping up with these appointments is even more critical.

Watch for Environmental Hazards If you work around chemicals or in an industrial setting, don't ignore the safety protocols. That protective gear might be uncomfortable, but it's there for a reason. Long-term exposure to certain chemicals can take a toll.

Building a Preventive Mindset

Preventing cancer isn't about living in fear. It's about maintaining your top form, being mindful of risks, and making informed decisions about your health. Every step you take to protect your body strengthens your defenses and gives you a better chance at staying healthy. Prevention is about stacking the odds in your favor, knowing that you're prepared, and taking control of what you can.

Taking care of yourself doesn't mean you're weak or paranoid. It means you're wise enough to understand that strength isn't just about muscles or endurance—it's about resilience. That means having a body that's ready for whatever gets thrown your way.

Final Thoughts on Prevention

Testicular cancer might not be something you can always prevent, but awareness and smart choices put you in a stronger position. Taking these steps doesn't guarantee anything, but it does stack the odds in your favor. Stay informed, keep tabs on your body, and don't shy away from taking action.

This isn't about obsessing over every risk; it's about staying sharp, staying strong, and being ready for anything. Knowing your risk factors and making a few smart adjustments can go a long way. So take charge, make the right moves, and stay ahead of the game. Being prepared isn't just smart—it's the foundation of real strength.

Part II: Navigating Treatment Options

Michael A's Journey: Fighting Back

At just 17 years old, Michael's world turned upside down. What was initially thought to be a hernia was revealed to be Stage 2B testicular cancer on March 26, 2010. The diagnosis came as a shock, and the fear was immediate. Michael described the moment as a nightmare. "Cancer meant death," he thought, and the idea of losing his life before it had truly begun was overwhelming. But Michael wasn't one to back down from a fight. Deep down, he resolved to face the battle head-on and not let cancer define his future.

Michael's treatment began with an orchiectomy on April 1. Unfortunately, the cancer had spread to lymph nodes in his abdomen, necessitating three intense rounds of inpatient chemotherapy—five days on, sixteen days off. The physical toll was grueling, with relentless nausea, fatigue, and feelings of isolation as his friends continued their lives while he endured hospital stays. Despite the challenges, Michael stayed determined and buoyed by the unwavering support of his family, friends, and the medical team at Cook Children's in Fort Worth. He credits his oncologist, Dr. Karen Albritton, and the compassionate staff for helping him find moments of light during a dark time.

Chapter 5

Treatment Options for Testicular Cancer

When you're up against a testicular cancer diagnosis, knowing your treatment options can make all the difference. Testicular cancer is highly treatable, especially when caught early, and there are three main ways to tackle it: surgery, radiation, and chemotherapy. Each treatment comes with its own approach, side effects, and purpose in the overall plan. Here's a straightforward look at each treatment type, what to expect, and how each one plays a role in getting you back on track.

Surgery: The First Line of Defense

For most guys, surgery is the first and often the most effective treatment for testicular cancer. It's a direct way to remove the cancer and reduce the chances of it spreading. The procedure most often used is called an orchiectomy, which involves removing the affected testicle. While it might sound intimidating, orchiectomy is one of the fastest and most reliable ways to contain the cancer.

Radical Inguinal Orchiectomy

A radical inguinal orchiectomy is the primary surgical procedure for testicular cancer. The surgeon makes an incision in the groin (inguinal region) to remove the affected testicle, which reduces the risk of spreading cancer cells into the scrotum or other parts of the body. While losing a testicle can be a heavy hit emotionally, many men choose to get a prosthetic implant. This option can help with body image and confidence after surgery.

Check Your Testosterone Before Surgery

Before undergoing orchiectomy, ask your doctor to test your baseline testosterone levels. This simple blood test provides a critical reference point for your hormonal health. While most men maintain normal testosterone production with one testicle, having your pre-surgery levels documented allows your medical team to monitor any changes and intervene quickly if needed accurately. If you later experience symptoms like fatigue, decreased libido, or mood changes, your baseline measurement becomes invaluable for determining whether hormone replacement therapy is necessary. Don't skip this step—knowing your starting point empowers you and your doctors to protect your long-term quality of life.

In most cases, men can still produce enough testosterone with one testicle, so hormone levels and sexual function typically aren't affected. However, if you notice any changes, hormone replacement therapy (HRT) is an option to keep everything balanced.

Lymph Node Surgery

If the cancer has spread beyond the testicle, another type of surgery may be necessary: retroperitoneal lymph node dissection (RPLND). This procedure removes lymph nodes in the back of the abdomen to prevent cancer from spreading further. RPLND is usually reserved for cases where the cancer has moved beyond the testicle, especially in non-seminoma cancers. Skilled surgeons focus on minimizing risks, especially to the nerves controlling ejaculation.

Open vs. Robotic RPLND: Understanding Your Options

RPLND can be performed through two distinct approaches: open surgery and robotic-assisted laparoscopic surgery. Open RPLND, the traditional gold standard, involves a single large abdominal incision that gives surgeons direct, unobstructed access to the retroperitoneal lymph nodes. This approach enables the most thorough lymph node removal, facilitates better handling of complex anatomy or bulky disease, and offers decades of proven outcomes at experienced centers. The tradeoff is a longer recovery time, more postoperative pain, and a larger scar. Robotic RPLND uses small incisions and specialized instruments controlled by the surgeon through a console, offering faster recovery, less pain, minimal scarring, and typically shorter hospital stays. However, robotic surgery requires highly specialized expertise, may not be suitable for all cases (particularly bulky or complex disease), and has a shorter track record with fewer long-term outcome studies. The choice between approaches depends on your specific cancer characteristics, your surgeon's expertise, and the experience of your center. At high-volume centers, both techniques can achieve excellent cancer control and nerve preservation—the surgeon's skill and experience matter more than the technique itself.

Skilled surgeons focus on minimizing risks, especially to the nerves controlling ejaculation.

Recovery from RPLND can take a bit longer than orchiectomy, with some soreness in the area, and requires a careful approach to avoid any damage to nearby nerves.

Radiation Therapy: Targeting Cancer Cells Directly

Radiation therapy is another effective method, especially for seminomas, which are highly sensitive to radiation. This treatment uses high-energy rays or particles to kill cancer cells by damaging their DNA.

External Beam Radiation Therapy (EBRT)

The most common form of radiation used for testicular cancer is external beam radiation therapy (EBRT). During EBRT, a machine outside the body directs radiation to the specific area where cancer cells are most likely to be hiding, usually the lymph nodes. This is typically done after surgery to catch any remaining cells that might have slipped through.

Radiation sessions are relatively short, often lasting 15–30 minutes each, but they're done multiple times a week for several weeks. Common side effects of EBRT include fatigue, skin reactions, and a temporary reduction in sperm count, which may affect fertility. It can take months or even years for sperm counts to return to normal, so if fertility is a concern, talk with your doctor about sperm banking before starting radiation.

Because radiation can slightly raise the risk of secondary cancers, regular follow-ups are essential for catching any future issues early.

Chemotherapy: Systemic Treatment for Cancer

When testicular cancer has spread beyond the initial area or poses a high risk of recurrence, chemotherapy steps in as a powerful option. Chemo works differently from surgery or radiation; instead of targeting a specific area, it's a systemic treatment. That means it travels throughout the body to hunt down cancer cells wherever they might be hiding.

Types of Chemotherapy Drugs

The most common chemo regimen for testicular cancer is a combination of cisplatin, etoposide, and bleomycin, known as BEP. This cocktail is known for its effectiveness, particularly for advanced stages or high-risk cases. The drugs are typically given in cycles, allowing the body to rest between treatments while the drugs continue to work.

High-Dose Chemotherapy and Stem Cell Transplant

In rare cases, when the cancer is aggressive or has come back, high-dose chemotherapy followed by a stem cell transplant might be an option. Here's how it works: doctors collect and freeze your own healthy blood-forming stem cells. Then, you're given high doses of chemo to knock out the cancer completely. Afterward, the stem cells are reintroduced to help your body recover and rebuild bone marrow. It's a serious treatment approach, usually reserved for when other options haven't worked, but it can offer a fighting chance in the most challenging cases.

What to Expect from Each Treatment Type

Each treatment type has a different approach and set of side effects, so here's a breakdown of what to expect:

Surgery Expectations and Side Effects

Recovery Time: Orchiectomy recovery is typically straightforward, with most men needing just a few days to a week of downtime.

Hormone Levels: If you're left with one testicle, it usually picks up the slack in testosterone production. But if there's any impact on hormone levels, hormone replacement therapy can keep things balanced.

Emotional Impact: Losing a testicle can feel like a major change, but remember, this is about eliminating cancer. Many men find confidence and peace of mind with a prosthetic implant, if that feels right for you. But there are a variety of factors that men need to consider before deciding which prosthetic is right for them.

With lymph node surgery, expect a longer recovery. Some soreness and restricted movement are normal. And, because the surgery is near the abdominal nerves, there's a risk (though rare) of affecting ejaculation.

Radiation Therapy Expectations and Side Effects

Session Length: Sessions are usually quick, around 15 to 30 minutes, but you'll have them multiple times per week over several weeks.

Side Effects: You may feel fatigued, and skin irritation in the treated area is common. Radiation can also temporarily reduce sperm count, so if having children is in your plans, consider sperm banking.

Long-Term Effects: Regular follow-ups are crucial, as radiation can slightly increase the risk of other cancers down the line.

Chemotherapy Expectations and Side Effects

Chemotherapy is known for its tough side effects, which vary widely from person to person, but it's effective. Here's what to expect:

Fatigue and Nausea: Feeling tired and nauseous is common, but anti-nausea meds can help.

Hair Loss: Not everyone loses hair, but it's a possibility. Just know it's temporary and part of the fight.

Fertility: Chemo can impact sperm production, so talk to your doctor about options like sperm banking if you're thinking about kids in the future.

Other Risks: Some drugs, like cisplatin, can impact kidney function and hearing, so your doctor will likely monitor these.

For high-dose chemo and stem cell transplants, expect a more intense experience with potentially stronger side effects. This treatment is reserved for more advanced or recurrent cases and often requires hospitalization and close monitoring.

Managing Side Effects and Recovery

Every treatment has side effects, but knowing how to handle them can make a huge difference.

Energy Levels: Fatigue is a reality with any cancer treatment, so listen to your body. Get rest when you need it, but try to keep moving to help maintain strength.

Fertility Concerns: Both chemo and radiation can impact fertility. If having kids is part of your future plans, discuss options like sperm banking with your doctor early on.

Mental Health: The physical battle is only part of the challenge. The emotional toll is real. Talking with a counselor or joining a support group can make a difference. The Testicular Cancer Foundation offers connections with other survivors, so don't hesitate to reach out.

Follow-Up and Long-Term Care

After treatment, you're not done. Follow-up care is just as important to make sure everything's still clear. Expect regular physical exams, blood tests to check for tumor markers, and imaging tests to keep an eye on any potential recurrence.

First Two Years: Plan on seeing your doctor every 3 to 4 months.

Years Three to Five: Visits usually decrease to every 6 months.

After Five Years: If everything's looking good, annual check-ups become the norm.

Final Thoughts on Treatment

Testicular cancer treatment is a serious fight, but it's also one that most men win. With options like surgery, radiation, and chemotherapy, you've got powerful tools to beat this. Each treatment has its pros and cons, and some side effects will have a greater impact than others. However, knowing what to expect helps you stay in control.

Whether you're just starting treatment or planning your recovery, stay informed, stay strong, and lean on the support around you. This is a fight you can win, and with the right approach, you'll come out on the other side ready for whatever's next.

Chapter 6

Surgical Treatments

When you're hit with a testicular cancer diagnosis, surgery is often the first line of attack. Surgery for testicular cancer is about one thing—getting the cancer out. From the initial tumor removal to complex lymph node surgeries, the goal is clear: eliminate the cancer while preserving as much function and quality of life as possible. In this chapter, we'll break down the types of surgical treatments, what to expect with each, and how they might impact fertility and sexual health.

Types of Surgeries and What to Expect

The main surgeries used to treat testicular cancer are radical inguinal orchiectomy and retroperitoneal lymph node dissection (RPLND). Here's the rundown on each procedure and what they bring to the table.

Radical Inguinal Orchiectomy

Most men facing testicular cancer start with a radical inguinal orchiectomy. In this surgery, the affected testicle is removed through a small incision in the groin. This approach is done intentionally—making the incision in the groin, instead of directly on the scrotum, helps to reduce the risk of cancer cells spreading during the procedure.

What to Expect During the Procedure: You'll be under general anesthesia, so you won't feel a thing. The surgeon makes a small cut in the groin, removes the cancerous testicle, and then seals up the incision. The surgery is straightforward and typically lasts less than an hour. Many guys go home the same day, making this a relatively quick and efficient procedure.

Recovery: Post-surgery, expect some soreness in the area. You'll need to avoid strenuous activity for a couple of weeks, but most men are back to their usual routines fairly quickly. Any discomfort fades as you heal, and before long, you're good to go. The scar is small and discreet, so it won't be a reminder of your cancer battle every time you look in the mirror.

Retroperitoneal Lymph Node Dissection (RPLND)

If there's a risk that cancer has spread beyond the testicle, you might be looking at a more complex surgery called retroperitoneal lymph node dissection (RPLND). In RPLND, the surgeon removes lymph nodes from the back of the abdomen, catching any stray cancer cells that might be lurking. This surgery is usually recommended if imaging or blood tests suggest the cancer could have spread.

Two Surgical Approaches

RPLND can be performed using two different techniques: open surgery or robotic-assisted laparoscopic surgery. Open

RPLND involves a larger abdominal incision and represents the time-tested gold standard, offering excellent visualization and the ability to handle complex cases, though with longer recovery time. Robotic RPLND uses small incisions and advanced technology for faster recovery and less scarring, but requires specialized expertise and may not be appropriate for all situations. Your surgeon will recommend the best approach based on the extent of your disease, their experience, and what your specific case requires. Both methods can be highly effective when performed by experienced surgeons at high-volume centers—the key is finding a specialist who has mastered their chosen technique.

What to Expect During the Procedure: RPLND is more complex than orchiectomy and requires a longer time under general anesthesia. The surgeon makes an incision along the abdomen to access and remove the lymph nodes. Because of its complexity, RPLND is usually done by specialists with a lot of experience in testicular cancer. After the surgery, you'll spend a few days in the hospital recovering.

Recovery: Recovery from RPLND takes more time—expect a month or two before you're back to full strength. Physical movement will be restricted for a while, and you'll need to avoid lifting heavy objects or doing intense physical activities. Despite the longer recovery, RPLND is a powerful option to help reduce the chance of cancer returning.

Impact on Fertility and Sexual Health

Surgery for testicular cancer isn't just about taking out the tumor—it can affect other parts of your life, particularly fertility and sexual health. Here's what you should know.

Fertility Concerns

With most testicular cancers, if only one testicle is removed (orchiectomy), the other testicle is usually enough to keep testosterone levels and sperm production in the normal range. The remaining testicle often steps up, ensuring your body has what it needs to function properly. However, some men may notice a dip in sperm count, and in cases where both testicles are removed (which is rare), fertility and testosterone production can be impacted significantly.

For guys looking to have kids down the road, sperm banking is an option worth considering. The process involves storing sperm before treatment begins, allowing you to preserve your options if surgery or additional treatments like chemotherapy affect fertility.

Retroperitoneal Lymph Node Dissection (RPLND) and Fertility

RPLND can affect fertility in a different way. The surgery is close to nerves that control ejaculation, so there's a chance of retrograde ejaculation, a condition where semen flows back into the bladder instead of out through the penis. While this doesn't impact the ability to have an erection or sexual pleasure, it can affect fertility. Most experienced surgeons perform a nerve-sparing RPLND to preserve these functions, but it's something to discuss with your doctor.

Testosterone Levels

Testosterone production typically remains stable with one testicle, so most men don't notice a change in muscle mass, mood, or libido. However, if there's a drop in testosterone levels, hormone replacement therapy (HRT) is an option. HRT can be administered in various ways, from injections to topical gels, ensuring you maintain energy, muscle tone, and overall well-being.

Prosthetic Testicles and Body Image

Losing a testicle can have an emotional impact. You might worry about how it looks or how it affects your masculinity. That's a normal reaction, and it's okay to feel that way. Many men opt for a prosthetic testicle, which looks and feels similar to a natural testicle. This can be a simple way to address any self-consciousness about the change, giving you one less thing to worry about.

Risks and Complications of Surgery

Like any surgery, these procedures come with some risks. Here's what you need to be aware of:

Infection: Any surgery carries a risk of infection. Your doctor will give you antibiotics to prevent this, and keeping the incision clean is important.

Bleeding and Blood Clots: Some bleeding is normal, but heavy bleeding or clotting can be an issue in more complex surgeries like RPLND. Your healthcare team will monitor for this.

Nerve Damage: With RPLND, there's a chance of nerve damage affecting ejaculation. Nerve-sparing techniques reduce this risk, but it's still a possibility. Talk to your surgeon about their approach to protecting these nerves.

Anesthesia Risks: General anesthesia is safe for most people, but it comes with some risks, especially for those with other health conditions. Discuss any concerns with your anesthesiologist.

Choosing the Right Surgeon

Picking the right surgeon is crucial, especially for something as specialized as testicular cancer surgery. Look for a surgeon with significant experience in these procedures, particularly RPLND. Don't be afraid to ask about their experience, how many similar surgeries they've done, and their complication rates.

It's also okay to get a second opinion. Finding a surgeon at a high-volume cancer center with a dedicated team often leads to better outcomes. If you're unsure, take the time to get another perspective—cancer surgery is a big deal, and you want to feel confident in your choice.

Preparing for Surgery and Recovery

A little preparation goes a long way toward a smooth recovery. Here are some tips:

Plan for Recovery: Arrange for time off work and help with chores. Surgery takes a toll, and you'll need some downtime to get back to full strength.

Pack Essentials: If you're having RPLND, plan for a hospital stay of a few days. Bring comfortable clothes, books, and anything that helps you pass the time.

Get Mentally Ready: Surgery can be nerve-wracking. Talking to other survivors or joining a support group can make a difference. Knowing that others have walked this path and come out strong can be a huge confidence boost.

Stay Active (Once You're Cleared): Once you're cleared by your doctor, get moving. Walking, light activity, and stretching can help with recovery and get you back on your feet faster.

Life After Surgery: Moving Forward

Surgery is a big step, but life goes on, and recovery is part of the journey. Here are a few things to keep in mind as you get back to normal:

Listen to Your Body: Recovery isn't a race. It's okay to push yourself, but know your limits. If you need rest, take it.

Check in with Your Doctor: Follow-up appointments are essential to monitor for recurrence. Stick to the schedule and stay in touch with your healthcare team.

Stay Active and Healthy: A healthy lifestyle makes a big difference. Regular exercise, a balanced diet, and avoiding tobacco and excessive alcohol can help keep you feeling strong.

Stay Connected: Lean on your support system, whether it's family, friends, or a support group. Going through cancer treatment is no small thing, and you're not alone.

Final Thoughts on Surgical Treatments

Surgery for testicular cancer is more than just a physical fight—it's a mental and emotional one too. Orchiectomy and RPLND each bring their own challenges, but they're tools to get you past cancer and back to living. The impact on fertility and sexual health can be managed, and there are options for sperm banking, prosthetics, and hormone therapy if you need them.

Remember, surgery is just one step in the journey. It's a powerful one, but with the right mindset and support, you'll come out stronger on the other side. You're not just a patient; you're a survivor, and each decision brings you closer to a cancer-free life. Stay informed, stay resilient, and keep moving forward—you've got this.

Zach's Summit: Conquering Stage 3 Testicular Cancer

In 2019, just two days before his 22nd birthday, Zach received a life-altering diagnosis: Stage 3 testicular cancer. "To say it's been a roller coaster is an understatement," he reflects. The shock was overwhelming, and while Zach struggled to process the news, his first instinct was to comfort his mom, who broke down in tears. "I told her it will all be okay," he recalls, not yet fully grasping the battle ahead.

Zach's treatment plan was intense—a combination of an orchiectomy, four cycles of BEP chemotherapy, and an open RPLND. It tested his mental and physical endurance, but Zach leaned heavily on his support system of friends, family, and faith to get through it. "I couldn't have done it without them," he says. Despite the challenges, he found ways to celebrate milestones along the way: halfway through chemo, the last day of treatment, and finally hearing the words "cancer-free."

One moment stands out among his victories. While undergoing treatment, Zach promised his girlfriend (now wife) that if he survived, they would climb a mountain in New Zealand. At the time, she didn't think much of it, but Zach was determined. Fast forward to nearly five years later, Zach kept his word. He flew to New Zealand with his wife and reached the summit of Roy's Peak, a journey that symbolized his triumph over cancer and his commitment to living fully. "It was a huge goal and accomplishment," he says with pride.

Chapter 7

Radiation Therapy

Radiation therapy is one of the main weapons in the fight against testicular cancer, especially when it comes to a type known as seminomas. While it might sound intense, radiation therapy is a powerful, targeted approach that focuses on wiping out any remaining cancer cells that surgery might have missed. This chapter breaks down how radiation therapy works, what you can expect during treatment, and the side effects you might face in both the short and long term.

How Radiation Therapy Works

Radiation therapy for testicular cancer uses high-energy X-rays or particles to destroy cancer cells. The goal is simple: kill off any cancer cells that might still be hanging around after surgery without harming too many healthy cells nearby. It's particularly effective for seminomas because this type of testicular cancer is highly sensitive to radiation.

External Beam Radiation Therapy (EBRT)

The most common type of radiation used for testicular cancer is External Beam Radiation Therapy (EBRT). Here's how it works:

Preparation and Planning Radiation therapy starts with a planning session, called simulation, where your healthcare team maps out exactly where the radiation should be directed. Using imaging scans (like CT or MRI), they determine the precise location to target, aiming at cancer-prone areas like lymph nodes near the testicles.

Treatment Process During treatment, a machine directs radiation beams from outside the body to the targeted areas. It's quick—you're usually in and out in about 15 to 30 minutes per session, with most of that time spent getting positioned correctly. The actual radiation exposure lasts only a few minutes. Radiation therapy is typically delivered multiple times a week for several weeks, depending on your specific treatment plan.

Precision and Control The radiation machine is incredibly precise, aiming the beams directly at cancer-prone areas to minimize exposure to surrounding healthy tissue. This controlled approach helps ensure that the treatment is effective while keeping side effects as low as possible.

What to Expect During Radiation Therapy

Radiation therapy is typically painless, so don't expect to feel anything during the actual treatment. However, as the sessions add up over time, you may start noticing some side effects. Everyone's body reacts differently, so what you experience might be mild or more intense, but knowing what to expect helps you stay prepared.

Fatigue Fatigue is one of the most common side effects of radiation therapy. The energy your body uses to repair healthy cells impacted by radiation can leave you feeling worn out. This tiredness often builds up over the course of treatment, so pace yourself and make sure to get plenty of rest. Staying hydrated, eating well, and doing light exercise like walking can also help combat fatigue.

Skin Reactions Because radiation is directed at a specific area on the body, you might notice skin reactions in the treated area. Skin can become red, irritated, or feel like a mild sunburn. Most of the time, these effects are mild and go away a few weeks after treatment ends. Your doctor can recommend specific creams to soothe the skin, but avoid any lotions or treatments that aren't approved by your healthcare team, as certain ingredients can make skin reactions worse.

Loss of Appetite and Nausea Some men experience mild nausea or a lack of appetite as a side effect. While it's not as common as with chemotherapy, it can happen, especially if radiation is directed near your abdominal area. Eating smaller meals more frequently and avoiding heavy, greasy foods can help manage these symptoms. If nausea becomes bothersome, your doctor can prescribe medication to help keep it in check.

Temporary Sperm Count Reduction Radiation therapy can temporarily lower your sperm count, which may affect fertility. For most men, this reduction is temporary, with sperm count returning to normal within a year or two. If you're concerned about future fertility, consider discussing sperm banking with your doctor before starting radiation. Banking sperm ensures you have options if family planning is part of your long-term goals.

Long-Term Impacts of Radiation Therapy

While radiation therapy is an effective way to reduce the risk of cancer returning, it's important to be aware of the potential long-term impacts. Here's what you need to know:

Fertility and Sperm Production For most men, sperm production returns to normal within a couple of years. However, in rare cases, sperm production might be permanently reduced, especially if higher doses of radiation were used. If fertility is a concern, sperm banking before starting radiation can provide a backup option.

Risk of Secondary Cancers Radiation therapy does increase the risk of developing secondary cancers later in life. These risks are generally low, but they're something to keep in mind. The benefit of eliminating the current cancer usually outweighs this risk, but regular follow-up appointments and monitoring will be part of your post-treatment care to keep an eye on your overall health.

Cardiovascular Health Studies have shown that men who undergo radiation therapy might have a slightly higher risk of developing cardiovascular issues over time, particularly if the radiation was directed near major blood vessels. This doesn't mean you're guaranteed to develop heart problems, but staying on top of your cardiovascular health with regular check-ups, a healthy diet, and exercise is a smart move.

Hormone Levels Radiation doesn't directly affect testosterone production unless both testicles are impacted, which is rare. In most cases, hormone levels remain steady, but if you do notice changes in energy, mood, or libido, bring it up with your doctor. Hormone replacement therapy (HRT) is available if you need it to keep your testosterone levels balanced.

Psychological Impact Radiation therapy isn't just a physical battle; it can take a toll mentally as well. The experience of going through cancer treatment and dealing with side effects can lead to feelings of anxiety or depression. Talking to a therapist or joining a support group can help you manage these emotions. Having a strong support system, whether it's friends, family, or a group of fellow survivors, can be incredibly grounding.

Managing Side Effects and Staying Strong

Radiation therapy might come with some challenges, but there are strategies to manage these side effects and stay strong throughout treatment.

Rest When You Need It: Fatigue can build up over time, so listen to your body. Rest when you need to, but don't hesitate to keep moving with light activities like walking, which can help fight off fatigue.

Take Care of Your Skin: Gentle, fragrance-free skin care products can help keep the treated area comfortable. Avoid scrubbing, wearing tight clothing, or exposing the treated area to extreme temperatures (hot or cold).

Nutrition and Hydration: Eating a well-balanced diet and staying hydrated can make a difference in your overall energy and well-being. If you're struggling with nausea, talk to your doctor, who can prescribe medications to help keep it under control.

Stay Connected: Keeping in touch with friends, family, or support groups gives you a solid emotional foundation. Lean on your support network to help you through the rough days.

Ask Questions: Don't hesitate to reach out to your doctor or care team about any side effects or concerns. Whether it's about managing fatigue, dealing with skin irritation, or understanding long-term risks, they're there to support you.

Looking Ahead: Life After Radiation Therapy

Once your radiation treatments are complete, it's time to focus on recovery and moving forward. Here are a few things to keep in mind post-treatment:

Follow-Up Appointments Regular follow-ups are essential to monitor for any signs of recurrence and manage any lingering side effects. Expect check-ups every few months for the first couple of years, which will gradually decrease in frequency over time if all looks good.

Healthy Lifestyle Choices Radiation therapy does increase some long-term risks, so taking care of your body is key. Focus on eating well, exercising regularly, and avoiding tobacco. Reducing alcohol intake can also help lower your risk for secondary health issues.

Mental Health Matters The impact of cancer treatment doesn't end when treatment stops. Many men find it helpful to stay in touch with support groups, a counselor, or other survivors who understand what they've been through. Cancer is a major life event, and processing it can take time.

Stay Informed Keep learning about testicular cancer, and don't hesitate to discuss new research or treatment options with your healthcare provider. Being proactive about your health is the best way to stay on top of any changes.

Final Thoughts on Radiation Therapy

Radiation therapy for testicular cancer is a powerful, targeted way to keep cancer from coming back. While the treatment itself is painless, the side effects and long-term impacts can be challenging. The key is to stay informed, communicate with your healthcare team, and listen to your body. Radiation therapy might bring some obstacles, but it's also a crucial step toward a cancer-free future.

Stay tough, stay informed, and take care of yourself throughout the journey. With the right mindset and support, you'll come through stronger on the other side, ready to take on whatever life throws your way.

Chapter 8

Chemotherapy

Chemotherapy is one of the most powerful tools in the fight against testicular cancer, especially when the cancer has spread beyond the testicle or poses a high risk of recurrence. Chemo targets cancer cells throughout the body, making it effective against cancer that surgery alone can't reach. In this chapter, we'll go over the main chemotherapy protocols for testicular cancer, what to expect from treatment, and how to manage side effects and recovery.

Chemotherapy Protocols

Chemotherapy for testicular cancer is often used alongside or after surgery, particularly when cancer has spread to lymph nodes or other areas. The main regimen used for testicular cancer combines three chemotherapy drugs: cisplatin, etoposide, and bleomycin (often called the BEP regimen). Here's what each drug does:

Cisplatin Cisplatin is a platinum-based drug that damages the DNA in cancer cells, making it harder for them to multiply. It's known for being highly effective against testicular cancer but also for its strong side effects, particularly nausea and kidney damage.

Etoposide Etoposide works by stopping cancer cells from dividing, which slows down their growth. It's often paired with cisplatin to increase the overall effectiveness of treatment.

Bleomycin Bleomycin targets the DNA in cancer cells, similar to cisplatin, but it's particularly effective at killing cells in their later stages. However, it comes with its own set of potential side effects, including lung toxicity, so doctors carefully monitor lung function during treatment.

Understanding the BEP Regimen

The BEP protocol is usually given in cycles, allowing your body to rest between treatments. A common schedule includes three to four cycles, with each cycle lasting about three weeks. During each cycle, you'll receive chemo drugs over several days, followed by a break before the next cycle begins.

Each cycle follows this general pattern:

Days 1–5: You'll receive a combination of cisplatin and etoposide daily. On Day 1, bleomycin is also given.

Days 8 and 15: Additional bleomycin treatments.

Your exact treatment plan may vary depending on your individual case, so talk with your oncologist to understand the details of your regimen.

What to Expect from Chemotherapy

Chemo isn't easy—it's a tough treatment that packs a punch. But being prepared for what's ahead can help you manage the experience.

During Treatment

Expect to spend several hours at the hospital or treatment center each day you receive chemo. You'll likely have a port placed in your chest to make the process easier and reduce the need for frequent needle sticks. A port is a small medical device surgically implanted under your skin, usually below your collarbone, with a catheter that connects directly to a large vein. Instead of starting a new IV each treatment, nurses access the port through your skin with a special needle, allowing chemotherapy drugs to flow directly into your bloodstream. This protects your smaller veins from damage, reduces discomfort, and makes each session more efficient. While you're receiving the drugs, you might feel fine, but the effects often kick in later in the day or within a few hours..

Most men start noticing side effects during the first few days of treatment. The intensity varies, but fatigue and nausea are common. Make sure to arrange for transportation to and from treatment if possible, as the fatigue can make driving difficult.

Short-Term Side Effects

Chemotherapy drugs are powerful, and they don't just affect cancer cells—they can also impact healthy cells, leading to side effects. Here are some of the most common side effects and how to handle them:

Fatigue Fatigue during chemo can be intense, making it tough to get through the day. Listen to your body, get as much rest as you need, and don't hesitate to lean on your support network. Light activity, like walking, can also help you feel more energized over time.

Nausea and Vomiting Chemo is notorious for causing nausea, but medications (called antiemetics) can help manage it. Take these meds as prescribed to stay ahead of nausea. Eating small, bland meals and avoiding rich or greasy foods can also help.

Hair Loss Hair loss is common with chemo, and it typically begins a few weeks after treatment starts. The good news is that it's temporary—your hair will grow back after treatment ends. Some men choose to shave their heads before hair loss starts, while others let it fall out naturally. Do what feels right for you.

Appetite Changes Many men lose their appetite during chemo, either due to nausea or changes in taste. Eating smaller, more frequent meals and drinking plenty of fluids can help. High-calorie, nutrient-dense foods can keep your energy up even if you're eating less.

Mouth Sores Mouth sores, or mucositis, can make eating uncomfortable. Avoid spicy, acidic, or crunchy foods, and rinse your mouth with a mild saltwater solution to soothe soreness. Your doctor can also prescribe a special mouthwash to help with the pain.

Low Blood Counts Chemotherapy can lower your blood counts, making you more prone to infections, anemia, and bruising. Avoid crowds and sick people to reduce your infection risk, and stay on top of handwashing and hygiene. If you notice symptoms like fever, chills, or unusual bruising, contact your healthcare provider immediately.

Managing Long-Term Side Effects

Chemotherapy is effective, but some side effects can linger even after treatment is over. Here's what to be aware of and how to manage long-term impacts.

Fertility Concerns Chemotherapy, particularly with cisplatin, can impact sperm production. While this is often temporary, it can be permanent for some men. Sperm banking before starting chemo is a wise option if you plan to have children in the future.

Hearing and Kidney Function Cisplatin can sometimes cause hearing issues (like ringing in the ears or hearing loss) and affect kidney function. Your doctor will monitor these closely, but stay alert to any changes and bring them up during your follow-up appointments.

Neuropathy Some men develop neuropathy (nerve damage), which causes tingling, numbness, or pain in the hands and feet. In most cases, neuropathy improves over time after treatment ends, but for some, it can be long-lasting. Physical therapy and medications can help manage symptoms if they persist.

Emotional and Psychological Impact Cancer treatment is physically demanding, but the emotional toll can be just as challenging. Chemo fatigue, the impact on fertility, and the ups and downs of treatment can lead to anxiety and depression. Many men find it helpful to connect with support groups or a therapist to process the experience. The Testicular Cancer Foundation and other organizations offer resources and connections with other survivors.

Recovery After Chemotherapy

Once your last chemo cycle is behind you, it's time to focus on recovery. Here's what to expect and how to get back on your feet:

Gradual Return to Normalcy After chemotherapy, your body will need time to bounce back. Energy levels will gradually improve, but give yourself time—recovery isn't a race. Focus on eating well, staying hydrated, and incorporating gentle exercise as you're able.

Follow-Up Appointments Regular follow-ups with your doctor are essential to monitor your recovery and watch for any signs of recurrence. You'll likely have blood tests and imaging scans at regular intervals in the months and years after treatment.

Building Strength Chemotherapy can take a toll on muscle strength, but getting back to an active lifestyle can help you rebuild. Start slow with light exercises, like walking or yoga, before transitioning to more vigorous activities as you regain strength.

Mental Health Check-Ins The mental impact of chemo is real, and it doesn't end just because treatment does. Check in with yourself regularly, and don't hesitate to seek counseling if you're struggling. Talking with other survivors who know the journey can also be incredibly helpful.

Tips for Handling Chemo Like a Pro

Chemo is a tough road, but there are ways to make the journey a little easier:

Stay Ahead of Nausea: Take your anti-nausea meds on schedule, even if you feel okay. Staying on top of nausea is easier than dealing with it after it starts.

Keep a Treatment Journal: Writing down symptoms, emotions, and side effects can help you and your doctor track what's working and what isn't. It's also a good way to see how far you've come.

Ask Questions: Don't hesitate to ask your doctor or chemo nurse about anything you're unsure of. The more you understand your treatment, the more in control you'll feel.

Final Thoughts on Chemotherapy

Chemotherapy is one of the hardest parts of dealing with testicular cancer, but it's also one of the most effective tools for beating it. Side effects are tough, but knowing what to expect and how to handle them gives you the upper hand. Take it one day at a time, lean on your support system, and remember that this treatment is a powerful step toward a cancer-free life.

You're tougher than chemo, and every cycle gets you closer to the end. Keep your eye on the goal, push through the rough days, and remember—you're fighting for a future that's worth every bit of this struggle.

IF THESE BALLS COULD TALK

Chapter 9

Follow-Up Care and Monitoring

Finishing treatment for testicular cancer is a huge milestone, but the journey isn't over. Regular follow-up care is crucial for keeping you on track and catching any signs of recurrence early. For many men, this follow-up period can bring peace of mind, but it can also come with its own set of anxieties. Knowing what to expect can make this part of the journey feel less daunting and help you feel confident about your long-term health. In this chapter, we'll cover the importance of follow-up care, what happens during these appointments, and how to stay proactive in maintaining your health.

The Importance of Regular Check-Ups

Follow-up care serves several key purposes after testicular cancer treatment:

Detecting Recurrence Early Testicular cancer has a high cure rate, especially if detected and treated early, but there's always a risk it could come back. Most recurrences happen within the first two years after treatment, making regular follow-ups essential for catching any changes as soon as possible. If cancer does return, finding it early gives you the best shot at beating it again.

Monitoring Side Effects Treatment can come with long-term side effects, some of which might not show up until months or even years later. Follow-up care helps your healthcare team monitor your health, manage any lingering side effects, and keep you feeling as strong as possible.

Supporting Mental and Emotional Health Cancer's impact isn't just physical—it can take a toll on your mental and emotional well-being, too. Follow-up appointments give you a chance to discuss any anxieties, mood changes, or stress you may be experiencing. Many men find that talking with their doctor or a counselor during these visits helps them manage the psychological side of recovery.

Guiding Long-Term Health Follow-up care helps set you up for a healthy future by checking in on all aspects of your health, not just cancer-related issues. Your doctor can guide you on lifestyle choices that can boost your health in the long run, including diet, exercise, and ways to reduce your risk of other health problems.

What to Expect During Follow-Up Visits

Your follow-up care plan will be customized based on your specific case, but it typically includes a combination of physical exams, blood tests, and imaging scans. Here's a breakdown of what to expect.

Follow-Up Schedule

The schedule for follow-up visits depends on the specifics of your diagnosis and treatment. Most men can expect appointments on this general timeline:

First Year After Treatment: Every 3 to 4 months

Second Year: Every 4 to 6 months

Years 3 to 5: Every 6 to 12 months

After 5 Years: Annual visits

If your doctor detects any issues during a check-up, they might increase the frequency of visits or request additional tests. The goal is to monitor your health closely during the period when recurrence is most likely and then gradually reduce the frequency if all remains well.

Physical Examinations

At each follow-up appointment, your doctor will perform a physical exam. They'll check for any lumps, swelling, or other abnormalities in your remaining testicle and nearby lymph nodes, as well as examine your abdomen. Physical exams help catch any early signs of recurrence and provide a chance to discuss any symptoms you've noticed.

Blood Tests

Blood tests are an essential part of follow-up care for testicular cancer. They're used to monitor tumor markers, which are substances that some types of cancer cells produce. High levels of these markers in the blood can indicate that cancer cells are present.

The primary tumor markers for testicular cancer are:

Alpha-Fetoprotein (AFP)

Human Chorionic Gonadotropin (HCG)

Lactate Dehydrogenase (LDH)

Not all types of testicular cancer produce tumor markers, so their importance depends on your specific case. If you had elevated tumor markers before or during treatment, your doctor will likely use these blood tests to monitor for recurrence.

Imaging Scans

Imaging tests are another key part of follow-up care, particularly if your cancer was advanced or had spread. Common imaging scans include:

Chest X-Rays: Testicular cancer can spread to the lungs, so regular chest X-rays help catch any signs of recurrence in that area.

CT Scans: CT scans provide a detailed view of your abdomen, pelvis, and chest. These scans are especially useful for monitoring lymph nodes and other areas where cancer could reappear.

Your doctor will decide the frequency and type of imaging based on your initial cancer stage and treatment plan. Imaging scans aren't typically needed as frequently as blood tests and physical exams, but they're crucial for providing a more detailed look when necessary.

Staying Proactive in Your Health

Follow-up care is a team effort, and you play a key role in staying on top of your health. Here are some ways to stay proactive:

Perform Regular Self-Exams Self-exams are still important, even after treatment. Regularly checking your remaining testicle for any lumps, swelling, or changes can help you catch any issues early. Knowing what feels normal can make it easier to recognize changes if they occur. Make it a habit to perform a self-exam every month.

Report Symptoms Immediately Don't wait for your next follow-up appointment if you notice something unusual. Symptoms like lumps, back pain, cough, shortness of breath, or any other unusual physical changes should be reported to your healthcare provider right away. These could be signs of recurrence or side effects that need attention.

Keep a Health Journal Many men find it helpful to keep a journal of their health, noting any symptoms, mood changes, or concerns that arise between appointments. A health journal can also be a useful tool to track your progress and any patterns that may emerge. Bringing your notes to follow-up appointments helps your doctor get a clear picture of how you're doing and any areas that need extra attention.

Ask Questions and Stay Informed Follow-up appointments are your opportunity to ask questions about your recovery, future health, and any concerns on your mind. If you have questions about your risk of recurrence, potential long-term effects, or lifestyle changes, don't hesitate to bring them up with your doctor. Staying informed helps you feel more in control of your health.

Managing Long-Term Effects of Treatment

Some side effects from testicular cancer treatment may linger, and follow-up care can help you manage these long-term impacts. Here are a few common long-term effects and how to address them:

Fertility If you've had chemotherapy, radiation, or an orchiectomy, fertility may be a concern. While many men retain their fertility after treatment, some experience a temporary or permanent reduction in sperm count. If you're considering starting or expanding your family, discuss fertility options with your doctor, who can refer you to a fertility specialist if needed.

Hormone Levels Losing a testicle can sometimes affect testosterone production, although most men with one testicle continue to produce enough. If you notice symptoms like low energy, mood changes, or a reduced sex drive, discuss these with your doctor. Testosterone replacement therapy can be an option if levels are low.

Psychological Impact Cancer recovery can come with feelings of anxiety, stress, or even depression. You've been through a lot, and processing it all can take time. If you're experiencing mental health challenges, talk to your doctor, who may refer you to a counselor, psychologist, or support group. Connecting with others who've been through the same experience can be incredibly beneficial.

Cardiovascular Health Some treatments, particularly radiation and certain chemotherapy drugs, can slightly increase your risk of cardiovascular issues. Make heart health a priority by eating a balanced diet, exercising regularly, avoiding tobacco, and limiting alcohol. Regular check-ups can help keep an eye on your cardiovascular health.

Life Beyond Cancer

Life after testicular cancer means finding a new normal. Follow-up care is an important piece of that puzzle, but so is focusing on what's next. Here are a few ways to move forward confidently:

Set Health Goals Think about setting health goals that go beyond cancer recovery. Whether it's building strength, eating better, or getting regular exercise, setting positive goals can keep you focused on the future.

Stay Connected Joining a support group or keeping in touch with fellow survivors can help you feel supported and understood. The Testicular Cancer Foundation and similar organizations provide networks where men can share their experiences and offer support to one another.

Embrace the New Normal Life after cancer can feel different, but it's a new chapter, and it's yours to shape. Follow-up care helps keep you healthy, but finding things that bring you joy, fulfillment, and purpose will help you thrive beyond recovery.

Final Thoughts on Follow-Up Care

Follow-up care isn't just about check-ups; it's about staying healthy and strong for the long haul. Regular appointments, self-care, and a proactive approach to your health help keep you on track and give you peace of mind. Cancer is a battle, but recovery is about rebuilding and moving forward.

With a solid follow-up plan, a strong support system, and a commitment to your health, you're setting yourself up for a long, healthy future. You've been through the hardest part—now it's time to focus on staying strong and embracing life beyond cancer.

Part III: Managing Life During and After Treatment

Jacob's Story: Finding Strength Through the Fight

Jacob's battle with testicular cancer came at a time when life was supposed to be coming together—his late 20s, right in the middle of finishing his college degree. The diagnosis hit him like a ton of bricks, bringing a wave of surgeries, treatments, and uncertainty. But through it all, he found something unexpected: a new perspective on life.

Initially, the gravity of his diagnosis didn't sink in. He recalls his doctor saying, "I'm sorry you're dealing with this," but at the time, it didn't fully register. All he knew was that his hormone levels were off and there was a mass in his testicle. The true weight of the situation dawned on him slowly, piece by piece, over the next several weeks.

Unlike many others, Jacob's journey started with a lymph node biopsy instead of an orchiectomy. Once the cancer was confirmed, he jumped headfirst into four grueling cycles of chemotherapy with etoposide and cisplatin, fighting the spread of tumors before eventually undergoing the orchiectomy. Even now, there's a question mark hanging over his treatment plan—whether he'll need an RPLND surgery down the road.

Receiving the biopsy results was the first time in weeks he felt like he could breathe again. The fear of dying had gripped him tightly, but finally knowing exactly what he was up against gave him clarity and a renewed sense of purpose. The support from his loved ones became his anchor, reminding him that he wasn't fighting alone.

IF THESE BALLS COULD TALK

Chapter 10

Mental Health and Emotional Well-Being

Getting hit with a cancer diagnosis isn't just a physical battle; it's a mental one, too. From the first moment you hear the words "you have cancer," your mind goes into overdrive. Anxiety, fear, anger, and even guilt—all of these emotions can hit you like a ton of bricks. You're not alone in feeling this way, and it's nothing to be ashamed of. In fact, facing cancer means dealing with one of the toughest mental challenges out there.

This chapter dives into the psychological impact of a cancer diagnosis, coping strategies to keep you steady, and resources to help you take control of your mental health. You've already proven your strength just by dealing with the physical side of cancer, but let's tackle the mental game, too.

The Psychological Impact of a Cancer Diagnosis

When you're told you have cancer, it can feel like the ground's been pulled out from under you. You're suddenly in a world of doctor's visits, treatment schedules, and tough decisions. That kind of pressure takes a toll on anyone's mental health.

Fear and Uncertainty It's normal to worry about the future. Will the treatment work? What will life look like down the road? Cancer is an uncertain journey, and the fear of the unknown can be tough to deal with. But here's the thing—fear doesn't have to run the show. Recognizing these worries is the first step to taking back control.

Anger and Frustration Cancer can feel like it's stolen something from you, whether it's your health, your time, or your peace of mind. Feeling angry about it isn't only normal—it's healthy. You didn't ask for this, and you've got every right to feel frustrated. Accepting that anger is part of the process can actually help you work through it and move forward.

Isolation and Loneliness One of the toughest parts of cancer is feeling like no one really gets what you're going through. Friends and family may be supportive, but they're not the ones sitting in the chemo chair or dealing with post-surgery pain. This sense of isolation is common, but it doesn't have to be permanent. Connecting with others who've been through the same experience can make all the difference.

Changes in Self-Image Cancer changes your body, and it can mess with how you see yourself. Surgery, hair loss, or even just the fatigue from treatment can make you feel like a different person. It's hard to feel like yourself when you're dealing with so much physical change, and it's normal to struggle with self-image as a result.

Survivor's Guilt Some men experience what's known as survivor's guilt, especially if they've seen others who didn't make it through similar battles. You might ask yourself, "Why did I survive when others didn't?" Survivor's guilt is common, but it doesn't mean you should feel guilty for making it through. You fought hard to survive, and that's something to be proud of.

Coping Strategies and Mental Health Care

The mental side of cancer requires as much attention as the physical side, and taking care of your mental health is a sign of strength, not weakness. Here are some strategies to keep your mind strong and steady during this journey.

1. Acknowledge Your Feelings

You've been through a lot, and it's okay to feel whatever you're feeling. Ignoring emotions or trying to "tough it out" can actually make things worse over time. Let yourself feel those emotions—anger, fear, sadness—and don't judge yourself for it. Emotions are part of the process, and accepting them helps you start moving forward.

2. Practice Mindfulness and Stay in the Present

Cancer tends to make you worry about the future, but focusing on what's in front of you can help ground you. Practicing mindfulness—whether it's through meditation, deep breathing, or even just taking a few minutes to focus on the here and now—can help lower stress and anxiety. Staying in the present keeps your mind from wandering down dark roads.

3. Set Small, Achievable Goals

When life feels overwhelming, breaking things down into small, manageable steps can make a big difference. These goals don't have to be massive; they can be as simple as taking a short walk, getting outside for a few minutes, or calling a friend. Each small win is a step toward regaining control, and over time, those steps add up.

4. Find Strength in Physical Activity

Physical exercise isn't just good for your body; it's great for your mind, too. Exercise can help improve your mood, increase energy levels, and give you a sense of accomplishment. You don't have to go all out at the gym—even light activities like walking or stretching can make a difference. Find something you enjoy, and make it part of your routine.

5. Connect with a Support Group

There's a unique comfort in talking with others who truly understand what you're going through. Support groups, whether in person or online, can be a safe space to vent, share experiences, and get advice from men who've been down the same road. The Testicular Cancer Foundation and similar organizations offer support groups that can help you feel less alone.

6. Consider Professional Help

Therapy or counseling isn't just for times of crisis—it's a powerful tool for anyone going through a tough experience. A trained mental health professional can provide strategies for managing stress, working through tough emotions, and finding strength in the face of uncertainty. Talking to a professional can offer a fresh perspective, and they can give you tools to handle whatever comes next.

7. Focus on What You Can Control

Cancer can make life feel unpredictable, but focusing on things within your control can help. Whether it's following a healthy diet, sticking to your treatment plan, or practicing good sleep habits, taking charge of the areas you can control gives you a sense of stability.

Building a Resilient Mindset

Resilience is about bouncing back, and going through cancer builds a kind of mental toughness that not much else can. Here's how to cultivate a mindset that keeps you moving forward, no matter what challenges you face.

Embrace the Journey

This might not be the road you'd planned to travel, but it's the one you're on. Accepting the journey—struggles and all—can help you make peace with it. Instead of focusing on "why me?" try shifting your mindset to "what now?" It's not easy, but finding meaning in the experience can help you come out of it stronger.

Lean on Your Support System

A strong support system is worth its weight in gold. Let friends, family, and loved ones help. It's okay to ask for support and let others be there for you. Whether it's a buddy to talk to, someone to go to appointments with, or just a friend to grab a beer with, connection is vital for staying mentally strong.

Celebrate Small Victories

Don't wait for the "big win" to celebrate. Every small step counts, whether it's making it through a treatment session, getting back to a routine, or just having a good day. Celebrate those moments—they're signs of progress, and they remind you that you're moving forward.

Focus on Gratitude

It might sound simple, but finding things to be grateful for can help shift your mindset. Even on tough days, look for something—anything—that you can appreciate, whether it's a friend's support, a good meal, or even just a few moments of peace. Gratitude doesn't ignore the hard stuff; it just helps balance it out.

Long-Term Mental Health and Moving Forward

The impact of cancer doesn't end when treatment does. Recovery is a marathon, not a sprint, and mental health care is just as important after treatment as it is during. Here's how to keep moving forward in the long haul.

Stay Connected with Support Resources Just because treatment ends doesn't mean you have to go it alone. Many men find support groups, counseling, or therapy helpful long after treatment. The Testicular Cancer Foundation and similar organizations offer ongoing support, so don't hesitate to reach out.

Focus on Rebuilding Your Life Cancer may have shaken things up, but now's the time to start rebuilding. Think about what matters most to you, and set goals that align with that. Whether it's getting back to work, pursuing a hobby, or spending more time with loved ones, focus on what makes you feel alive.

Give Yourself Grace Recovery isn't always a straight line. There may be good days and tough days, and that's okay. Be patient with yourself and remember that it's normal to need time to get back to feeling like yourself.

Continue Practicing Self-Care Self-care isn't a one-time fix; it's a lifelong practice. Keep taking care of your mind and body with regular exercise, a balanced diet, and sleep. These habits help keep you grounded and give you the energy to tackle whatever comes your way.

Final Thoughts on Mental Health and Well-Being

Taking care of your mental health through cancer and recovery isn't a luxury—it's essential. You're in the fight of your life, and keeping your mind strong helps you stay resilient, grounded, and ready to face whatever challenges come your way. Remember, you don't have to face this alone, and reaching out for support is a sign of strength.

You've already shown what you're made of. Now it's about building a mindset that helps you thrive in the long run. Stay tough, stay grounded, and keep moving.

IF THESE BALLS COULD TALK

Chapter 11

Navigating Conversations with Your Employer

When you're diagnosed with cancer, breaking the news to family and friends is challenging enough, but bringing it up at work? That's a whole other level. Navigating this conversation with your employer can feel overwhelming, but handling it with preparation and confidence is key to ensuring you get the support and accommodations you need. This chapter dives into practical strategies for having that conversation, understanding your legal rights, and making sure your workplace has your back through treatment and recovery.

Preparing for the Conversation

The more prepared you are, the easier it will be to discuss your diagnosis with your employer. Start by gathering all relevant details about your diagnosis, treatment plan, and how both may impact your work.

1. Gather Essential Information

Knowing the details about your diagnosis and treatment plan gives you a strong foundation when discussing your needs. Key information to collect includes:

Diagnosis: Understand the type and stage of your cancer.

Treatment Plan: Know your treatment schedule, the expected duration, and any anticipated side effects.

Work Impact: Consider how treatment might affect your ability to work, including possible absences, physical limitations, and necessary accommodations.

2. Plan Your Approach

Think through the best way to approach this conversation. Factors to consider:

Timing: Pick a time when you and your employer can have an uninterrupted discussion.

Setting: A private setting is best to allow for an open conversation about personal health.

Support: Bringing along a trusted colleague or HR representative can help if it makes you feel more comfortable.

Having the Conversation

When you sit down with your employer, honesty and directness are your best allies. Here's how to handle the conversation with clarity and confidence.

1. Start with the Facts

Begin by outlining the key aspects of your diagnosis and treatment plan. It's important to be clear, concise, and professional. For example, you might say, "I've recently been diagnosed with testicular cancer and will be undergoing treatment that may require time off for appointments and recovery."

2. Discuss How It Will Affect Your Work

Next, address how your treatment may impact your job duties. This could include absences, limitations on certain tasks, or a reduced schedule. By being transparent, you help your employer understand your needs and set clear expectations.

3. Request Specific Accommodations

If you need adjustments to your workload or schedule, don't be afraid to ask. Common accommodations might include:

Flexible hours

Remote work options

Adjusted workloads or deadlines

Physical accommodations, like a quieter workspace or more comfortable seating

4. Emphasize Your Commitment

Reassuring your employer that you remain committed to your responsibilities can help ease any concerns they may have about your performance. Acknowledge the challenges of balancing work with treatment, but express your determination to continue contributing to the team as best as possible.

5. Offer Documentation

Providing documentation from your healthcare provider can clarify your needs and substantiate your requests. This may include a note outlining your diagnosis, treatment plan, and any specific accommodations that might aid your recovery and well-being at work.

Understanding Your Rights

Navigating the workplace during cancer treatment isn't just about conversations; it's also about knowing your legal rights and protections. In the U.S., there are several laws that provide workplace protections for people facing serious health conditions.

1. Family and Medical Leave Act (FMLA)

The Family and Medical Leave Act (FMLA) allows eligible employees to take up to 12 weeks of unpaid leave for serious health conditions, including cancer. This leave can be taken all at once or intermittently (in smaller blocks), depending on your treatment needs.

FMLA ensures that your job is protected while you're on leave, meaning your employer can't fire or replace you because of your health condition. To qualify, you generally need to have worked at your company for at least a year and have logged at least 1,250 hours over the past 12 months.

2. Americans with Disabilities Act (ADA)

The Americans with Disabilities Act (ADA) requires employers to provide reasonable accommodations to employees with disabilities, which can include those undergoing cancer treatment. This law protects you from discrimination and ensures that your workplace makes necessary adjustments to support you during treatment. Reasonable accommodations could be anything from modifying your work hours to allowing remote work or making physical adjustments to your workspace.

3. Company Policies

In addition to federal laws, it's important to understand your company's specific policies on medical leave, sick days, and accommodations. Many companies have their own guidelines or programs in place to support employees facing medical challenges. Take the time to review your employee handbook, and don't hesitate to speak with your HR department for clarification.

Maintaining Open Communication

After that initial conversation, staying connected with your employer throughout your treatment is essential. Regular updates can help them manage your workload, adjust accommodations as needed, and plan ahead.

1. Keep Your Employer in the Loop

As treatment progresses, be proactive in communicating any changes in your condition, treatment schedule, or work capacity.

This doesn't mean you have to give daily updates, but providing a heads-up on significant changes helps everyone plan more effectively. If you anticipate needing additional accommodations or adjustments to your workload, don't wait to speak up.

2. Addressing Employer Concerns

Some employers may worry about your ability to meet deadlines or handle certain tasks. Be open to discussing these concerns and work together to find solutions that support both your health and the team's needs. This might involve adjusting deadlines, delegating specific tasks, or finding alternative ways to manage responsibilities.

3. HR and Employee Assistance Programs (EAPs)

Don't overlook your HR department or Employee Assistance Programs (EAPs). These resources can provide guidance on workplace accommodations, legal rights, and even mental health support. Many companies also offer counseling services, which can be helpful if you're feeling stressed or overwhelmed.

Navigating Workplace Support Systems

Beyond HR, there are other support networks and resources to help you stay balanced during this time. Tapping into these networks can offer not only practical advice but also emotional support.

1. Peer Support and Cancer Networks

Connecting with other cancer patients and survivors who've faced similar challenges can be a powerful source of support. The Testicular Cancer Foundation and other organizations provide platforms where individuals share experiences and strategies for balancing work with treatment. Support networks can offer advice, encouragement, and a sense of community that's invaluable during this time.

2. Friends and Trusted Colleagues

If you're comfortable, confide in a few trusted coworkers who can offer additional support. These colleagues can be helpful allies in the workplace, checking in on you, offering help when needed, and keeping you connected to the team.

Legal Protections and What to Do If Issues Arise

Most employers are supportive and understanding, but if you feel you're being treated unfairly or face discrimination due to your diagnosis, know that you have options.

Consult HR If you feel your employer isn't providing reasonable accommodations or is being unsupportive, bring the issue to HR. They're there to advocate for you and can help mediate any issues.

Seek Legal Advice if Necessary If the situation escalates or you believe your rights are being violated, you may want to consult with a legal professional who specializes in employment law. Organizations like the Equal Employment Opportunity Commission (EEOC) can also provide guidance on filing complaints and understanding your rights.

Final Thoughts on Workplace Conversations

Talking about cancer with your employer isn't easy, but being upfront and clear about your needs can set the tone for a supportive work environment. Remember, your health comes first, and you have every right to the accommodations that make your treatment and recovery as smooth as possible.

This conversation might be tough, but tackling it head-on shows your resilience and commitment. By preparing, understanding your rights, and staying proactive, you can make sure you have the support you need to keep moving forward, both at work and in your fight against cancer.

Rowan's Story: Finding Strength Through Community

Rowan's testicular cancer diagnosis at 27 turned his world upside down. A routine ultrasound revealed a mass, and within a day, he underwent a right radical orchiectomy. Three months later, he faced an open RPLND surgery. Physically, he recovered well, but mentally and emotionally, it was a different story.

As a father of two young children, facing his own mortality was overwhelming. Thoughts of recurrence, how his family would manage, and the fear of not being there for his kids weighed heavily on him. The emotional strain took a toll, making him distant from his loved ones. The reality of his diagnosis truly hit when his doctor recommended the RPLND—suddenly, it all felt undeniably real.

For weeks, Rowan struggled, feeling isolated despite the support of his family. Then, in 2018, his wife convinced him to attend the TCF Summit, and that decision changed everything. Initially hesitant, he found himself surrounded by men who understood his journey in a way no one else could. Meeting fellow survivors gave him the sense of connection and hope he had been missing.

Hearing the words that his RPLND pathology was clear brought immense relief, but it still took him a year to feel somewhat normal again. However, thanks to TCF and the camaraderie it provided, Rowan found new perspectives and a sense of healing he hadn't thought possible.

IF THESE BALLS COULD TALK

Chapter 12

Managing Feelings of Isolation

Cancer doesn't just take a toll on the body; it can make you feel like you're cut off from the world. Treatment routines, physical symptoms, and emotional ups and downs can create a sense of isolation that's hard to shake. Feeling disconnected is common for cancer patients, especially when the people around you can't fully grasp what you're going through.

Why This Book Goes Deep on Mental Health

Most testicular cancer resources focus exclusively on medical treatment—the surgeries, the staging, the survival rates. But surviving cancer isn't just about killing cancer cells. The psychological impact of a testicular cancer diagnosis carries unique weight: you're often young, in what should be your prime, facing a disease that strikes at the core of your identity as a man. The isolation, the fear, the questions about fertility and masculinity—these aren't minor side effects. They're central to your experience and your recovery. Yet they're rarely discussed with the same urgency as treatment protocols. This book refuses to treat your mental and emotional health as an afterthought. Your psychological survival matters as much as your physical survival, and addressing isolation isn't optional—it's essential.

This chapter is all about tackling those feelings head-on. We'll explore strategies to keep you connected and supported, emphasizing the power of support groups and networks. There's strength in numbers, and reaching out to others who understand can make all the difference in facing the mental and emotional challenges that come with cancer.

Understanding Why Isolation Happens

Isolation doesn't always mean being physically alone. It can also be a mental or emotional feeling, a sense of separation from those around you. Here are a few reasons why cancer can create these feelings of isolation:

Physical Limitations and Fatigue Treatment can sap your energy, making it tough to go out and spend time with people. Even simple social gatherings can feel like too much to handle when you're exhausted, leaving you spending more time at home and less with others.

Lack of Understanding from Others Cancer is hard to understand unless you've been through it. Friends and family may offer support, but they might not fully grasp what it's like to live with the physical and emotional side effects of treatment. This lack of understanding can make you feel distant, even from those closest to you.

Self-Consciousness and Changes in Self-Image Physical changes, like hair loss or weight fluctuations, can make it hard to feel confident or comfortable around others. It's normal to feel self-conscious about these changes, but isolating yourself often makes things worse.

Emotional Strain and Fear Cancer can bring fear and anxiety that others might not understand, and this emotional strain can feel like a heavy weight. Expressing these fears may feel difficult, and bottling them up can lead to feeling even more alone.

Strategies to Stay Connected and Supported

Isolation is a tough feeling to combat, but there are ways to break through it. Staying connected doesn't have to mean taking on a lot at once. Here are some practical ways to keep yourself feeling supported and connected, even on tough days.

1. Make Use of Digital Connections

When going out feels like a chore, technology can be a lifeline. Staying connected through texts, video calls, and social media helps maintain relationships without requiring too much energy. Reaching out to friends and family online can make you feel less isolated, even if you're spending more time at home. Join online groups, follow cancer support pages, or even schedule regular virtual coffee chats with friends.

2. Let Friends and Family In

Letting others in isn't always easy, but it's essential. Be honest with those close to you about what you're feeling. Tell them when you need support and how they can help. You don't have to put on a brave face all the time. Sometimes, just having someone to listen makes all the difference.

Don't hesitate to let friends and family know that even a quick text or message can make a positive impact. Sometimes, small gestures go a long way in reminding you that you're not alone in this journey.

3. Get Involved in Support Groups

Support groups bring together people who truly understand what you're going through. Whether you join in-person or online, these groups provide a space where you can share your experiences, ask questions, and connect with others who are facing similar challenges.

Support groups offer many benefits:

Shared Understanding: There's something powerful about talking to people who "get it." Knowing others are walking a similar path can reduce feelings of isolation.

Practical Advice: Group members often share tips for managing side effects, handling stress, or even recommendations on what to bring to chemo. This kind of practical advice is invaluable.

Emotional Support: A support group is a safe place to talk about feelings that might be hard to express elsewhere. You can vent, share fears, or celebrate small wins without worrying about how it sounds.

Check with organizations like the Testicular Cancer Foundation, which offers resources to connect you with in-person or virtual support groups.

4. Consider One-on-One Counseling

Therapists and counselors specialize in helping people deal with isolation, anxiety, and other challenges that cancer brings. Speaking with a mental health professional gives you a chance to talk openly about your feelings in a private, judgment-free space. They can provide personalized strategies to handle isolation and help you find ways to feel connected, even during tough times.

Don't hesitate to ask your healthcare team for a recommendation if you're interested in finding a therapist who specializes in cancer care. Some therapists even offer telehealth sessions, so you can attend appointments from home.

5. Build a Routine That Keeps You Engaged

Creating a daily or weekly routine with a few activities you enjoy can add some structure to your life and give you something to look forward to. Whether it's reading, watching a favorite show, gardening, or even cooking a new recipe, having a few "constants" can make you feel more connected to life outside of cancer.

If possible, include some form of physical activity in your routine. Even light exercise, like walking, can help boost your mood, keep you energized, and make you feel more engaged. Plus, getting outside can help combat feelings of isolation by connecting you to the world around you.

6. Explore Hobbies That Foster Connection

Hobbies can help you stay engaged and even connect with others. If you enjoy activities like cooking, photography, or writing, consider joining a class or sharing your work online. Many communities are built around shared interests, and participating in these spaces can help you feel less isolated. You could join a virtual class, start an Instagram page for your photography, or join an online book club—whatever feels right for you.

7. Reach Out to Cancer-Specific Networks

Organizations like the Testicular Cancer Foundation provide resources specifically designed for those dealing with cancer. These networks offer a unique kind of support, connecting you to people who understand the specific challenges of testicular cancer. They can also help you find educational resources, survivor networks, and local or online events to keep you involved in the cancer support community.

The Importance of Support Groups and Networks

There's real strength in numbers. Being part of a support group or network can remind you that you're not alone, and it can also provide a sense of purpose. Whether you're joining an online forum, attending an in-person meeting, or even just following survivor stories on social media, these groups have a big impact on mental and emotional well-being.

1. Feeling Less Alone

When you're surrounded by people who understand your experience, it's a lot harder to feel isolated. Support groups bring together people who know what it's like to face cancer, and that shared understanding is powerful. You'll find that even just hearing others' stories can make you feel connected, especially on days when the isolation feels overwhelming.

2. Learning from Shared Experiences

Group members often share their experiences, advice, and personal stories. Hearing how others handle certain challenges, side effects, or emotional hurdles can give you practical ideas for managing your own journey. You'll pick up insights you may not get from doctors or friends who haven't walked this path.

3. Building New Friendships

A support group can be a place to meet people you'd otherwise never cross paths with, people who "get it" on a level that's hard to find elsewhere. These relationships can be incredibly valuable, offering a sense of camaraderie and trust that helps you through the highs and lows of treatment and recovery.

4. Gaining Strength from Survivor Stories

Many support groups and networks share survivor stories, which can be a huge boost when you're feeling low. Hearing about others who've made it through similar experiences can be incredibly motivating and provide hope that life can continue beyond cancer.

Final Thoughts on Combating Isolation

Isolation is tough, and it's normal to feel separated from the world when you're dealing with cancer. But there are tools, resources, and connections out there to help you break through that isolation. Staying connected doesn't mean you have to constantly be social—it means finding ways to feel supported, understood, and engaged, even if you're taking things one small step at a time.

Don't hesitate to reach out, whether it's to a friend, a support group, or an online community. By taking even a few small steps to connect with others, you'll find that isolation doesn't have to define your experience with cancer. Remember, you're not alone in this journey, and there's a world of support waiting to lift you up.

Chapter 13

Recovery After Successful Treatment

Making it through cancer treatment is an incredible milestone, but recovery doesn't end when the last session of chemo or radiation wraps up. After treatment, your body and mind both need time to heal, adjust, and rebuild strength. Recovery from cancer is a process, one that involves physical, mental, and emotional aspects, and it requires patience and commitment. This chapter offers insights into what to expect in your recovery journey, practical tips for rebuilding your strength, and how to navigate the new normal post-treatment.

Physical Recovery After Treatment

Cancer treatment, whether it's surgery, chemotherapy, or radiation, takes a toll on your body. After months of battling cancer, your body needs time to bounce back. Physical recovery looks different for everyone, depending on the type of treatment you had, your overall health, and any side effects you might still be dealing with.

1. Managing Fatigue and Rebuilding Stamina

Fatigue is one of the most common aftereffects of cancer treatment. It's a type of tiredness that isn't fixed by sleep and can last for months. Managing fatigue takes time, but there are strategies that can help:

Pace Yourself: Start small and work your way up. Gentle exercise like walking can be an effective way to gradually build back stamina.

Rest When You Need It: Listen to your body and don't push yourself too hard. Short naps or breaks throughout the day can help manage fatigue.

Establish a Routine: Set a daily routine that includes periods of rest and activity. It's all about finding a balance that works for you.

2. Nutrition and Hydration

Your body has been through a lot, and now it's time to fuel it right. A well-balanced diet can play a huge role in how you feel as you recover.

Prioritize Protein: Protein helps repair and rebuild tissues, making it especially important during recovery. Include lean meats, fish, eggs, beans, and nuts in your diet.

Stay Hydrated: Drinking enough water is crucial, especially if you're still dealing with side effects like dry mouth from radiation. Aim for plenty of water each day, and consider other hydrating options like herbal teas or water-rich fruits.

Add Nutrient-Dense Foods: Incorporate plenty of fruits, vegetables, whole grains, and healthy fats into your meals. These foods can help boost your immune system and give you the energy you need to regain your strength.

3. Regaining Muscle and Strength

Long periods of inactivity or side effects from treatment can cause muscle loss. Physical therapy or exercise is key to getting back into shape and regaining strength.

Start Slowly: Begin with gentle activities that don't strain your body, like walking, stretching, or yoga.

Build Up Gradually: Over time, add in light weight lifting or resistance training to rebuild muscle. Always go at your own pace, and don't rush the process.

Consider Physical Therapy: A physical therapist can design a safe and effective exercise program that's tailored to your needs. They can help you with balance, coordination, and flexibility exercises, which are all important during recovery.

4. Addressing Long-Term Physical Effects

Some side effects, like neuropathy (numbness or tingling in the hands and feet) or lymphedema (swelling due to lymph fluid buildup), may persist after treatment. If you're dealing with long-term side effects, work closely with your healthcare team or physical therapist to manage them. There are exercises and treatments that can help reduce symptoms and improve your quality of life.

Emotional Recovery After Treatment

The end of treatment can bring a lot of relief, but it can also stir up complex emotions. Some people feel anxious about the possibility of recurrence, while others feel lost or even depressed. Emotional recovery is just as important as physical recovery, and finding ways to take care of your mental health is a big part of your journey forward.

1. Processing Your Emotions

Going through cancer treatment is a life-changing experience, and it's normal to feel a mix of emotions when it's over. You may feel a sense of relief, gratitude, sadness, or even anger. Take time to acknowledge these feelings without judging yourself.

Talk About It: Opening up to friends, family, or a therapist can help you work through your feelings. You don't have to keep everything bottled up; sharing your experience can be incredibly healing.

Write It Out: Some people find comfort in journaling, where they can reflect on what they've been through and what they're feeling now. Writing down your thoughts can give you perspective and help you process your journey.

2. Dealing with Anxiety and Fear of Recurrence

One of the biggest challenges after treatment is dealing with the fear that cancer might come back. This fear is common, and while it may not go away entirely, there are ways to manage it.

Focus on the Present: Try not to let fear steal your focus from the here and now. Meditation and mindfulness exercises can help you stay grounded and centered.

Set a Follow-Up Plan with Your Doctor: Knowing that you'll have regular check-ups and monitoring can give you peace of mind. Have a clear follow-up plan in place so you know when to expect future appointments.

Consider Counseling: A mental health professional can help you manage anxiety and give you strategies for dealing with any worries about recurrence. Counseling can be a safe space to address these fears head-on.

3. Finding a New Normal

Life after cancer may not be exactly as it was before, and that's okay. This is a chance to rebuild on your own terms, to focus on what matters most to you.

Set New Goals: You might have goals you put on hold during treatment. Now is the time to think about what you want to pursue moving forward, whether it's personal projects, hobbies, or spending time with loved ones.

Redefine Your Priorities: Going through something as challenging as cancer often brings a new perspective on life. Let this experience shape your priorities and help you focus on what truly matters to you.

The Role of Rehabilitation and Physical Therapy

Physical therapy can be a game-changer in your recovery process, helping you rebuild strength, mobility, and confidence after treatment. Rehabilitation isn't just about physical recovery; it can boost your mental and emotional resilience, too.

1. Strengthening Muscles and Improving Mobility

Physical therapy often starts with exercises to regain muscle strength and improve range of motion. A physical therapist can help you with exercises specifically designed to target areas that may have weakened during treatment.

Functional Movements: Physical therapists focus on exercises that mimic daily activities, so you can gradually get back to a normal level of physical function.

Strength Training: As you progress, your therapist may add strength training to help build muscle and improve endurance. This can be especially important if you have lost muscle mass during treatment.

2. Addressing Treatment-Related Side Effects

Physical therapy can also help manage side effects like neuropathy, lymphedema, and balance issues. Therapists have specific techniques to help reduce pain and improve circulation, which can ease these symptoms.

Neuropathy Exercises: If you're dealing with tingling or numbness in your hands or feet, your therapist can show you exercises that improve blood flow and help reduce discomfort.

Lymphedema Management: For those dealing with lymphedema, a therapist can teach you lymphatic drainage techniques and exercises to reduce swelling and maintain range of motion.

3. Building Confidence and Restoring Independence

One of the biggest benefits of physical therapy is the confidence boost it provides. Each step forward in strength and mobility reminds you that you're reclaiming control over your body and your life.

Progress Tracking: Seeing improvements, no matter how small, can be motivating. Physical therapists often track your progress, so you can see your gains over time.

Supportive Environment: Physical therapists are trained to support your recovery at every step. They provide encouragement, guidance, and reassurance, which can make the process feel less intimidating.

Staying Connected with Support Systems

Support doesn't end when treatment does. Staying connected to family, friends, or support groups is a big part of recovery.

Lean on Your Support System: Friends, family, and even coworkers can provide comfort and companionship during recovery. Don't be afraid to reach out when you need someone to talk to or spend time with.

Join a Survivorship Group: Many cancer organizations offer groups specifically for people in recovery. These groups can provide camaraderie, shared experiences, and valuable insights from others who've been through similar experiences.

Final Thoughts on Recovery

Recovery is a journey, not a sprint. Take it one day at a time, and celebrate each small victory along the way. Be patient with yourself, set realistic goals, and stay open to support from others. By focusing on both physical and emotional healing, you're setting yourself up for a strong, healthy future.

You've come this far—now it's time to move forward, rebuild, and embrace life after treatment.

IF THESE BALLS COULD TALK

Chapter 14

Sexual Health and Relationships

Cancer treatment doesn't just affect the body—it can also have a big impact on your relationships and intimacy. When you're dealing with the aftereffects of surgery, chemo, or radiation, it's normal to feel like your body isn't quite the same. These treatments can impact everything from your energy levels to your body image, and even your sexual health. On top of that, there's the challenge of communicating openly with your partner, especially when it comes to sensitive topics.

This chapter is about facing these changes head-on. We'll look at how cancer treatment can impact sexual health, ways to adapt and maintain intimacy, and the importance of open communication with your partner. Cancer might bring new challenges to your relationship, but with honesty, support, and patience, you can navigate this part of recovery together.

Understanding the Impact of Treatment on Sexual Health

Cancer treatments like surgery, chemotherapy, and radiation can affect your sexual health in various ways. The changes you experience depend on the type of treatment you had, as well as any side effects you're dealing with post-treatment. Here's a breakdown of how different treatments can impact sexual health:

1. Surgery and Physical Changes

For many men with testicular cancer, surgery is the first step in treatment. An orchiectomy (removal of one testicle) is the most common surgical approach, and while it doesn't usually impact testosterone levels if only one testicle is removed, it can still affect how you feel about your body.

Body Image: Losing a testicle may lead to concerns about appearance and masculinity. While the change may not be visible to others, it's normal to feel self-conscious or to need time to adjust to your new body.

Prosthetics: Some men choose to get a testicular prosthetic to maintain a similar appearance to before surgery. It's a personal choice, and if it helps you feel more confident, it can be worth discussing with your doctor.

2. Chemotherapy and Hormonal Changes

Chemotherapy can take a toll on your energy levels, stamina, and libido. The physical exhaustion that comes with chemo can leave you feeling drained, both physically and mentally. Chemo may also affect hormone levels, leading to changes in sexual desire.

Reduced Libido: It's common for men to experience a drop in sex drive during and after chemotherapy. This can be temporary, but it might take time to return to previous levels of desire.

Sperm Production: Chemotherapy can also impact fertility by affecting sperm production. Many men choose to bank sperm before starting treatment to preserve their options for future family planning.

3. Radiation Therapy and Sensitivity Issues

Radiation can affect the nerves and tissues in and around the treatment area. Depending on where radiation is focused, it might lead to changes in sensation, which can impact sexual pleasure.

Nerve Sensitivity: If radiation affects nerves in the pelvis or abdomen, it can alter sensitivity and sometimes result in discomfort during intimacy.

Testosterone Levels: Radiation can sometimes impact testosterone production, leading to lower levels of the hormone. This may lead to fatigue, reduced libido, and other symptoms associated with low testosterone. Your doctor can test and monitor your hormone levels and may suggest hormone replacement therapy if needed.

Rebuilding Confidence and Body Image

Cancer treatment changes your body, and those changes can take time to accept. The first step in reclaiming confidence is to be patient with yourself. Healing is a process, and adjusting to physical changes requires time and self-compassion.

1. Give Yourself Permission to Heal

It's okay if intimacy doesn't feel the same as it did before treatment. Take things one step at a time, and allow yourself to heal physically and emotionally. You've been through a lot, and it's normal to need time to adjust.

2. Focus on What Makes You Feel Good

Your body has been through the ringer, so it's essential to focus on activities that make you feel good about yourself. This could be exercise, hobbies, spending time outdoors, or anything that gives you confidence and a sense of strength. Feeling good in your own skin can go a long way in restoring confidence in the bedroom, too.

3. Talk to a Counselor

If you're struggling with body image or self-esteem after treatment, consider speaking with a counselor. Mental health professionals can provide valuable tools and support, helping you work through complex emotions and build confidence.

Maintaining Intimacy and Connection with Your Partner

Open communication is key to maintaining intimacy. Cancer doesn't just affect you; it affects your partner, too, and it's essential to talk openly about the changes you're experiencing. Being honest can ease concerns, reduce misunderstandings, and help both of you adapt to this new phase together.

1. Talk Openly About How You're Feeling

Be honest with your partner about how treatment has impacted you, both physically and emotionally. Share any concerns or insecurities you might have, whether it's related to body image, fatigue, or changes in sexual desire. Open conversations help your partner understand where you're coming from and give them the chance to support you fully.

2. Take Things Slow and Keep It Simple

Intimacy doesn't have to be rushed. Take your time, and don't put pressure on yourself to get back to "normal" right away. Focus on small, simple gestures of closeness—holding hands, cuddling, or simply spending quality time together. Physical intimacy can take many forms, and sometimes starting slow is the best way to rekindle a connection.

3. Redefine Intimacy Beyond Physical Connection

Sexual intimacy is just one aspect of a relationship. Emotional intimacy—the deep connection you share with your partner—can be strengthened during challenging times like this. Try to focus on ways to connect emotionally, such as sharing your feelings, spending quality time together, or engaging in activities you both enjoy.

4. Be Patient with Yourself and Your Partner

Recovery is a journey, and patience goes a long way. Be kind to yourself, and don't rush the process. Your partner is also adjusting to changes, so giving each other space to process can make things easier. Remember, intimacy may look different after cancer treatment, and that's okay. Adapting to a "new normal" doesn't mean that connection or passion are out of reach.

Practical Tips for Rebuilding Sexual Health and Intimacy

Getting back to feeling comfortable and confident in the bedroom takes time, and small steps make a big difference. Here are some practical tips to help ease the transition back to intimacy:

1. Prioritize Comfort and Relaxation

Stress and anxiety can make intimacy feel even more challenging. Creating a comfortable, relaxed atmosphere can help you feel more at ease. Whether it's taking a warm shower beforehand, dimming the lights, or playing music, find ways to make the experience feel less stressful.

2. Focus on Foreplay

If you're worried about changes in sensation or stamina, focusing on foreplay can take some of the pressure off. Foreplay helps foster connection and build closeness without putting the focus solely on performance. It's an opportunity to explore what feels good and rebuild intimacy in a gradual, comfortable way.

3. Consider Consulting a Specialist

Some doctors and therapists specialize in sexual health and can offer guidance on how to manage changes in sexual function after cancer treatment. These specialists can provide practical advice and suggest exercises or techniques that may help. Don't hesitate to ask your healthcare team for a referral if you're interested.

4. Explore Products That May Help

Certain products, like lubricants or even erectile aids, can make intimacy more comfortable. If dryness or sensitivity is an issue, a good lubricant can make a significant difference. For more severe issues, medications or other aids are options worth discussing with your doctor.

The Importance of Patience and Adaptability

Adjusting to changes in sexual health and intimacy takes patience, both with yourself and with your partner. You may not get back to where you were immediately, and that's okay. Building a new normal might take time, but each small step counts.

Seeking Support from Other Survivors

If you're struggling with issues related to sexual health or intimacy, connecting with other cancer survivors can help. Many men have faced the same challenges, and hearing how others navigated these changes can provide encouragement, ideas, and reassurance. Support groups and survivor networks are great places to share experiences and get advice from people who truly understand what you're going through.

Final Thoughts on Sexual Health and Relationships

Recovering from cancer is about more than just physical health. Relationships, intimacy, and self-confidence are all important aspects of life that deserve attention and care. Take things at your own pace, be patient with yourself and your partner, and remember that you don't have to tackle this alone. Talking openly with your partner, reaching out for support, and exploring ways to adapt can help you build a strong, fulfilling relationship after treatment. Cancer may have changed some things, but it doesn't have to change the connection and closeness you share with your partner.

Daniel's Story: Facing the Fight Head-On

When Daniel was diagnosed with bilateral seminomas at 34, it hit him hard. The idea of losing something so personal and vital weighed heavily on him, but having a solid support system made all the difference. Family and friends surrounded him, offering comfort and distraction in the tough moments. The fear of what his diagnosis could mean was compounded by the rarity of his case—his doctors initially suspected other forms of cancer before confirming testicular cancer. Once the diagnosis was set, his biggest concern shifted from survival to how he would look and feel post-surgery. Fortunately, his wife's unwavering support reassured him that his worth wasn't defined by physical changes.

Daniel's first orchiectomy came a month after his ultrasound, a period filled with fear and uncertainty. The thought of hormone therapy loomed over him, but he focused on potential positives—hitting the gym and rebuilding his strength. When tests showed he was still producing enough testosterone, he felt a renewed sense of hope and opted for a partial orchiectomy instead of full removal. It was a rare choice, but one that allowed him to hold off on hormone therapy for as long as possible.

IF THESE BALLS COULD TALK

Chapter 15

Fertility and Family Planning

Cancer treatment can bring a lot of changes, and one of the areas it might impact is your ability to have kids down the line. For a lot of guys, especially younger men, fertility is a big part of thinking about the future. Cancer treatments like chemotherapy, radiation, and surgery can all affect fertility in different ways, and it's normal to feel concerned or even frustrated by that reality.

This chapter is all about tackling those concerns head-on. We'll break down how testicular cancer treatment can affect fertility, the options you have to preserve it, and the steps you can take to make sure you have choices when it comes to family planning. The goal is simple: to help you understand your options, feel more prepared, and take control of your future.

Understanding How Cancer Treatment Affects Fertility

The impact of cancer treatment on fertility depends on the type of treatment you're getting. Each treatment works differently, and some can have temporary effects, while others might lead to more permanent changes. Let's dive into how each type of treatment might affect fertility.

1. Surgery and Its Impact on Fertility

For many men with testicular cancer, the first step is surgery to remove one of the testicles—a procedure called an orchiectomy. If you've only had one testicle removed, the remaining one can still produce sperm and testosterone, which means fertility might not be affected at all.

However, if both testicles are removed, you won't be able to produce sperm naturally anymore. In cases like these, banking sperm before surgery becomes even more important. If you're in a situation where both testicles need to be removed, talk to your doctor about fertility preservation before surgery.

2. Chemotherapy and Sperm Production

Chemotherapy is designed to kill cancer cells, but it doesn't just target those cells—it can also impact sperm cells, which divide quickly, making them more vulnerable to chemo's effects. While some men regain fertility after chemo, others may face longer-lasting effects. Here's what to know:

Temporary Effects: For some men, chemo may cause temporary infertility. It might take months or even years for sperm production to return to normal.

Permanent Effects: Certain chemotherapy drugs are more likely to cause permanent infertility. It all depends on the specific medications and dosages used. If you're considering having kids in the future, talk to your doctor about the drugs being used and how they may impact fertility.

3. Radiation Therapy and Sperm Health

Radiation therapy can also affect fertility, especially if it's directed at the pelvic or abdominal area. Radiation can damage sperm production in the testicles, sometimes leading to infertility. In some cases, the effects are temporary, but higher doses can lead to permanent changes.

Shielding: If only one testicle is affected, doctors might be able to shield the other to minimize exposure to radiation.

Low vs. High Dose: The higher the radiation dose, the higher the risk of infertility. Ask your medical team about your specific radiation plan and the risks involved.

Options for Fertility Preservation

For guys who want to keep their options open for starting a family down the line, there are a few solid ways to preserve fertility before you start treatment. The good news? With the right steps, you can protect your ability to have kids later.

1. Sperm Banking

Sperm banking is one of the most common and effective methods for fertility preservation. The process is simple and straightforward: you provide a sperm sample that's frozen and stored until you're ready to use it.

Why It Works: Sperm can be safely stored for years without any decline in quality, so if you're thinking about having kids in the future, this is a solid option.

How It's Done: Typically, you'll go to a sperm bank or fertility clinic, where you'll give several samples over a few days. These samples are then frozen for future use.

2. Testicular Sperm Extraction (TESE)

If sperm production is low or you're not able to bank sperm before treatment, a procedure called testicular sperm extraction (TESE) may be an option. This involves a minor surgery where doctors remove a small sample of tissue from the testicle to look for viable sperm.

When It's Used: TESE is usually done if standard sperm banking isn't an option. It's also sometimes used for men who have undergone treatment and are now infertile but may still have some sperm in their testicular tissue.

Considerations: It's a more invasive option than sperm banking, but for some men, it's a valuable alternative if they want biological children down the line.

3. Hormone Preservation

If your cancer treatment involves lowering or blocking testosterone levels, there are ways to protect hormone health that can also indirectly support fertility. Hormone therapy is less about directly preserving sperm and more about keeping overall reproductive health intact, especially if low testosterone is an issue.

Testosterone Replacement Therapy: After treatment, some men might need testosterone replacement to maintain normal hormone levels. This isn't directly tied to fertility, but it can help maintain muscle mass, mood, and energy levels.

4. Fertility Counseling

Fertility counseling may not be a physical procedure, but it's one of the most important steps you can take. Speaking with a fertility specialist can help you understand all your options, weigh the pros and cons, and make a plan that feels right for you.

Know Your Options: A fertility specialist can guide you through every method, answer your questions, and help you create a plan for preserving fertility.

Planning for Parenthood: If you have a partner, counseling can help you both get on the same page, address concerns, and build a plan for the future.

Making Decisions for Your Future

The decision to preserve fertility isn't an easy one. It's personal, and it's about planning for a future that may feel uncertain at times. However, understanding your options and planning ahead can give you the freedom to make decisions for yourself and your future family. Here's how to approach this process with confidence:

1. Talk Openly with Your Doctor

Your healthcare team should be a trusted source of information and support. Don't hesitate to bring up any questions or concerns you have about fertility. Remember, it's your future on the line, so get clear answers on how your treatment may impact fertility and what steps you can take to protect it.

2. Discuss Your Options with Loved Ones

Fertility preservation is a big decision, and it's okay to lean on your loved ones for support. If you have a partner, talk to them about what you're considering, and make this decision together if it affects both of you. If you're making this choice solo, reach out to family or close friends who can provide input or simply listen to your thoughts.

3. Weigh the Costs and Benefits

Banking sperm, consulting specialists, or undergoing procedures like TESE all come with costs, both financial and emotional. Be sure to consider both the short-term and long-term impacts of each option. If you're worried about costs, ask your doctor or counselor about any financial assistance programs for cancer patients looking to preserve fertility.

Moving Forward with Confidence

Choosing to preserve fertility is a powerful step in planning for the future, but it's also just one part of the bigger picture. Fertility preservation gives you options, which can provide a sense of control in a time when it may feel like you don't have much control at all. It's about creating possibilities for yourself—so that, down the line, you have choices and the freedom to decide what's right for you.

What to Expect After Treatment: Fertility Testing

After treatment, some men may find that their fertility returns naturally over time, while others may need to revisit options like hormone therapy or even fertility treatments to grow their family. Here's what you can expect:

Regular Testing: Some doctors recommend follow-up fertility testing after treatment to check sperm counts and hormone levels. This can give you a clearer idea of where things stand.

Consult with a Fertility Specialist: If you're interested in starting a family, a fertility specialist can guide you through additional testing and help you decide on the best course of action.

Final Thoughts on Fertility and Family Planning

Cancer treatment may have thrown you a curveball, but it doesn't have to take your choices or your future. Preserving fertility is about giving yourself options so that, when the time comes, you can still make choices about family planning and parenthood. Take this part of your journey one step at a time. Ask questions, make informed choices, and don't hesitate to seek support along the way.

Cancer may be a part of your story, but it doesn't define every chapter. With knowledge and preparation, you can face this part of recovery with the same strength and resilience that got you through treatment. You've got a future to look forward to—now it's time to build it.

Part IV: Support Systems and Resources

IF THESE BALLS COULD TALK

Chapter 16

Comprehensive Support Systems

Dealing with testicular cancer is more than just a physical battle—it's an emotional, mental, and financial one, too. Facing a diagnosis, navigating treatment, and moving forward all require a solid support network. The Testicular Cancer Foundation (TCF) is here to provide that network, offering resources and support for both patients and their families every step of the way.

The Importance of Support Systems

When you're going through something as challenging as cancer, having a strong support system is crucial. That support might come from family and friends, healthcare providers, or organizations dedicated to helping cancer patients. Whether it's a listening ear, financial guidance, or practical help, a good support system can make all the difference.

Finding Community with TCF

One of the best ways to find comfort and strength during this time is to connect with others who understand what you're going through. TCF offers several ways for patients and caregivers to find community and support:

1. Online Support: Discord Community and Weekly Zoom Calls

The TCF Discord community is an online space where patients and survivors can come together, share their stories, and offer each other advice and encouragement. It's a space to find understanding and camaraderie. Additionally, TCF hosts weekly Zoom calls every Thursday at 7 PM CST. These virtual meet-ups provide a way to stay connected and share experiences in a supportive environment.

2. In-Person Events: Annual Summit and Regional Meetups

If you prefer face-to-face support, TCF holds an Annual Summit where patients, survivors, and caregivers can gather for a weekend of education and community building. This event offers a chance to connect with others, gain new insights, and find inspiration. TCF also organizes regional meetups for more localized support, allowing patients and families to connect closer to home.

Resources for Managing Financial and Practical Challenges

Cancer treatment can be costly, and the expenses often add up quickly. TCF understands the financial strain that testicular cancer can cause and offers resources and guidance to help patients and families manage these challenges.

Support for Caregivers

Caregivers play a vital role in the support system for individuals undergoing cancer treatment. Being a caregiver is rewarding, but it can also be incredibly challenging. TCF offers resources specifically for caregivers, helping them understand the journey, manage their own well-being, and provide the best possible support for their loved ones.

1. Caregiver Support Resources

TCF provides a caregiver guide that offers practical advice on how to care for someone with testicular cancer. It covers everything from understanding treatment options to managing daily responsibilities and finding support for themselves.

2. Self-Care for Caregivers

Taking time to care for oneself isn't just a luxury—it's necessary. TCF encourages caregivers to practice self-care, connect with support groups, and lean on resources when they need a break. Caregivers play a vital role, and maintaining their own health and well-being is crucial.

Prioritizing Emotional and Mental Health

Dealing with cancer can be emotionally overwhelming for both patients and families. TCF emphasizes the importance of mental health and offers a range of resources to help patients and caregivers cope.

Counseling and Support Services

Talking to someone who understands the emotional toll of cancer can be incredibly helpful. TCF offers access to counseling and mental health resources, providing a safe space for patients and families to process their experiences and find support.

Mindfulness and Self-Care Techniques

Incorporating mindfulness practices into your daily routine—like deep breathing or spending time in nature—can make a difference. These small acts of self-care are simple ways to reduce stress and support mental and emotional well-being.

Final Thoughts on Building a Support System

The road through cancer treatment isn't easy, but you don't have to go through it alone. TCF provides a range of support systems designed to meet the needs of patients, survivors, and caregivers alike. Whether you're looking for financial guidance, mental health support, or simply a community that understands, TCF is there to help. By reaching out and tapping into these resources, you'll be better prepared to navigate this journey and face each day with strength and confidence.

Chapter 17

The Role of Family and Friends

A cancer diagnosis is never a solo journey. While it primarily impacts the person diagnosed, the ripple effects touch everyone close to them—family members, friends, coworkers, and even distant relatives. The role of family and friends during this time is crucial, not only for the practical support they can provide but also for the emotional strength they can offer. Involving loved ones in the journey creates a web of support that can make a significant difference in the patient's ability to face the challenges ahead.

How Family Members Can Provide Support

Family members often find themselves as the front-line supporters, offering help in a variety of ways. While the specifics will vary depending on the person's needs and circumstances, these key areas of support can make a profound impact:

Offer Practical Assistance: Cancer treatment often comes with logistical challenges—doctor's appointments, managing medications, maintaining a home, and dealing with day-to-day responsibilities. Family members can step in by coordinating schedules, driving to appointments, preparing meals, or taking care of children or pets. For example, organizing a meal train or arranging for household cleaning services can alleviate stress for both the patient and their caregivers. These seemingly small acts of service can provide immense relief during an overwhelming time.

Be Present: Sometimes, the most important thing family members can do is simply be there. Presence isn't about always knowing the right thing to say; it's about offering companionship and reassurance. Whether it's sitting in silence during a difficult moment, holding their hand during chemotherapy, or just watching a favorite TV show together, these acts remind the person battling cancer that they are not alone. Presence provides comfort in ways words often cannot.

Encourage Open Communication: Creating a safe space for open and honest communication is vital. Patients may struggle with feelings of fear, anger, or hopelessness, and being able to express these emotions without judgment is crucial. Active listening—where the focus is on understanding rather than offering solutions—can help loved ones feel heard and validated. This builds trust and helps the patient feel less isolated in their journey.

Respect Their Wishes: Every cancer journey is deeply personal, and the choices patients make—whether about treatment, lifestyle changes, or how they spend their time—are theirs alone. Family members must respect these decisions, even if they differ from what they might have chosen. Offering support without overstepping boundaries is a delicate balance, but it's a necessary one to maintain trust and dignity.

Provide Emotional Stability: Cancer can be emotionally destabilizing, not just for the patient but for their entire family. Family members can help ground their loved ones by staying positive without being dismissive of the challenges. A steady and calm presence can provide a sense of security, especially during moments of uncertainty or fear. Reminders of hope, faith, and resilience can be especially powerful.

Educate Yourself: Understanding the type of cancer, the treatment process, and its potential side effects can help family members empathize more effectively and anticipate needs. It also shows commitment and solidarity, reassuring the patient that they are not facing this battle alone.

The Importance of Involving Loved Ones in the Journey

Including family and friends in the cancer journey isn't just beneficial for the patient—it strengthens the support network as a whole. Here's why it matters:

Shared Burden, Shared Strength: Involving loved ones creates a shared sense of purpose. When the physical and emotional load is distributed, the patient feels less isolated, and supporters feel empowered knowing they are contributing to the healing process. Families often report that working together in times of crisis brings them closer.

Promotes Healing Through Connection: Emotional connection is a powerful tool for healing. When patients feel surrounded by love and support, it can boost their mental and emotional state, which is a crucial component of overall well-being. Simple gestures like a heartfelt card, a phone call, or a visit can have a profound impact.

Strengthens Relationships: The journey through cancer often deepens bonds. Challenges have a way of bringing people closer, and families and friends frequently find that the shared experience of facing adversity creates lasting emotional ties.

Prevents Caregiver Burnout: Caregivers, often the closest family members, can experience significant stress. When friends and extended family step in, it eases the burden on primary caregivers. Sharing tasks like grocery shopping, babysitting, or simply sitting with the patient gives caregivers much-needed respite and reduces the risk of burnout.

Encourages the Patient to Keep Fighting: Knowing that others are invested in their journey can be a motivating factor for the patient. The love and support of family and friends remind them that they are not fighting for themselves alone but for the people who care deeply about them.

Practical Ways to Involve Loved Ones

Create a Support Plan: Coordinating care and support can feel overwhelming, but a clear plan makes it manageable. Assign tasks based on strengths—someone who enjoys cooking can prepare meals, while a tech-savvy family member can research treatment options or organize a GoFundMe for medical expenses.

Host Family Meetings: Regular updates and open discussions ensure everyone stays informed about the patient's needs, treatment progress, and any new challenges. These meetings also allow for honest conversations about how family members can best support the patient and each other.

Invite Participation in Key Moments: Whether it's joining a medical appointment, attending a support group, or celebrating milestones like the end of a treatment cycle, these moments create connection and build memories that reinforce the importance of togetherness.

Express Gratitude: Patients can involve loved ones by showing appreciation for their efforts. A simple "thank you" or acknowledgment of their help can go a long way in maintaining morale. Similarly, family members should express gratitude toward each other, fostering a spirit of collaboration and mutual respect.

Leverage Technology: For loved ones who live far away, technology bridges the gap. Regular video calls, texts, and emails can keep them involved and connected, ensuring that distance doesn't prevent meaningful participation.

A Word to Friends

Friends often want to help but may hesitate, fearing they'll overstep or say the wrong thing. If you're a friend of someone battling cancer, remember that your support matters. Reach out with offers of specific help—like driving them to appointments or picking up groceries—rather than general offers like, "Let me know if you need anything." The latter, while well-meaning, places the burden of asking for help on the patient.

Friends also play a unique role in providing a sense of normalcy. Talking about shared interests, reminiscing about happy memories, or engaging in activities unrelated to cancer can give the patient a much-needed mental break from the disease.

A Final Thought

The journey through cancer is not one anyone chooses, but it is one no one should face alone. Family and friends are an integral part of the process, providing the love, strength, and hope that make the fight more bearable. By leaning on their support and allowing them into the journey, patients can experience not just healing but the profound beauty of shared humanity. Together, they can find light even in the darkest moments and create a tapestry of love and resilience that will remain long after the battle is over.

Michael K's Story: Running the Race

Michael was 41 when he received a testicular cancer diagnosis, just a week after completing his first half marathon. The pain and discomfort he felt in his left testicle seemed like a lingering race injury, and despite finding a lump, he waited nearly three months before seeking medical advice. Fortunately, the cancer was still at Stage I, but Michael learned an important lesson: when something feels off, don't wait—get it checked out.

Initially, Michael believed testicular cancer was a "young man's disease" and never thought it would affect him in his 40s. He was nervous about what the diagnosis would mean, particularly regarding treatment options like chemotherapy or radiation. Thankfully, he had a supportive wife and a solid group of friends, including two men who had faced their own battles with cancer. They provided a roadmap and reassurance as he navigated the uncertainty. That support became even more crucial a year later when scans revealed the cancer had spread, and he needed a retroperitoneal lymph node dissection (RPLND).

The news of cancer growth was a gut punch. Surveillance had been his preferred route, avoiding harsher treatments, but now surgery was unavoidable. With the help of an experienced surgeon, Michael found hope in hearing the word "cure" as the goal. The surgery, though daunting, proved to be a success—no signs of cancer were found in the removed lymph nodes.

TESTICULAR CANCER FOUNDATION

Chapter 18

Legal Rights and Workplace Accommodations

Receiving a cancer diagnosis is life-changing, and managing treatment alongside everyday responsibilities can be overwhelming. For many, navigating legal protections and workplace accommodations becomes an essential part of the journey. Understanding your rights and the resources available can ease the burden and ensure that you're supported during this challenging time.

Legal Protections for Patients

Laws are in place to protect individuals diagnosed with cancer and other serious health conditions. These legal safeguards ensure that patients are not discriminated against and have access to necessary accommodations to manage their condition. Below are some key legal protections that may apply:

The Americans with Disabilities Act (ADA): The ADA prohibits discrimination against individuals with disabilities, including those diagnosed with cancer, in the workplace and other public spaces. Under the ADA:

Employers with 15 or more employees are required to provide reasonable accommodations unless doing so causes undue hardship.

Reasonable accommodations may include adjusted work hours, remote work options, additional breaks, or a temporary reassignment of duties.

The Family and Medical Leave Act (FMLA): The FMLA allows eligible employees to take up to 12 weeks of unpaid, job-protected leave within a 12-month period for serious health conditions. This law applies to:

Employers with 50 or more employees within a 75-mile radius.

Employees who have worked for the company for at least 12 months and logged 1,250 hours in the previous year.

This leave can be taken continuously, intermittently, or on a reduced schedule, depending on the patient's needs.

State and Local Laws: Many states have additional protections that may offer benefits beyond those provided by federal laws. For example, some states provide paid family leave, short-term disability benefits, or expanded job protections for those with serious illnesses.

The Genetic Information Nondiscrimination Act (GINA): GINA protects individuals from discrimination based on genetic information, including predisposition to certain cancers. Employers and insurance providers cannot use genetic information to make decisions about hiring, firing, or coverage.

Health Insurance Portability and Accountability Act (HIPAA): HIPAA ensures that personal health information is protected and cannot be disclosed without consent. This means that employers and colleagues cannot access your medical information unless you choose to share it.

Navigating Workplace Challenges

Balancing work responsibilities with cancer treatment can be physically and emotionally taxing. However, by understanding your rights and effectively communicating with your employer, you can find a path that works for your unique situation.

1. Disclosing Your Diagnosis

Deciding whether and when to disclose your cancer diagnosis to your employer is deeply personal. While there is no legal obligation to disclose unless requesting accommodations, open communication can foster understanding and make it easier to get the support you need.

Consider the following when disclosing your diagnosis:

Prepare in Advance: Before approaching your employer, understand your needs and the accommodations you'll be requesting. Gather information about your treatment schedule and potential side effects that might impact your work.

Involve Human Resources: HR professionals are trained to handle sensitive matters and can guide you through the process while maintaining confidentiality.

Be Honest, But Boundaries Matter: Share only as much as you're comfortable with. Focus on how your condition affects your work and what accommodations would help you perform your job effectively.

2. Requesting Workplace Accommodations

Workplace accommodations are modifications or adjustments that enable you to perform your job despite your condition. Under the ADA, reasonable accommodations might include:

Flexible work schedules to accommodate treatments or recovery time.

Remote work or hybrid arrangements.

Physical changes, such as an ergonomic workstation or a private space for rest.

Adjusted responsibilities, such as delegating physically demanding tasks.

To request accommodations:

Document Your Needs: Obtain a note from your healthcare provider outlining your condition and the accommodations required.

Submit a Written Request: While verbal requests are valid, a written request creates a clear record. Include details about your diagnosis (if you're comfortable sharing) and specific accommodations.

Collaborate with Your Employer: Work together to identify solutions that balance your needs with the organization's capabilities.

3. Managing Stigma and Bias

Unfortunately, some individuals face stigma or bias in the workplace after disclosing their diagnosis. To address these challenges:

Know Your Rights: If you experience discrimination, document incidents and consult your HR department or an employment attorney.

Educate Colleagues: Sometimes stigma stems from misunderstanding. If you're comfortable, share information about your condition to foster awareness and empathy.

Seek External Support: Cancer support groups or legal advocacy organizations can provide guidance and reassurance.

4. Financial Considerations

Cancer treatment often brings significant financial strain, and understanding your workplace benefits can help mitigate these challenges:

Short-Term and Long-Term Disability Insurance: If your employer offers disability insurance, it can provide partial income replacement during treatment or recovery.

Employee Assistance Programs (EAPs): Many companies offer EAPs, which provide free counseling, financial planning, or other resources for employees facing personal challenges.

Flexible Spending Accounts (FSAs) or Health Savings Accounts (HSAs): These accounts allow you to set aside pre-tax dollars for medical expenses, reducing out-of-pocket costs.

5. Transitioning Back to Work

If you take a leave of absence, returning to work can feel daunting. Planning ahead and easing into the transition can help:

Communicate Your Needs: Discuss any ongoing accommodations you may require with your employer.

Ease Back Gradually: If possible, start with part-time hours or lighter responsibilities before resuming your full workload.

Give Yourself Grace: Recovery takes time, and it's okay to acknowledge that you may not perform at your previous capacity immediately.

Resources for Legal and Workplace Support

There are numerous organizations and resources to help patients understand their legal rights and workplace protections. Consider reaching out to:

Cancer and Careers: A nonprofit that provides tools, training, and resources for working people with cancer.

The Equal Employment Opportunity Commission (EEOC): Offers information about your rights under the ADA and guidance on filing a discrimination complaint.

Local Legal Aid Organizations: Many communities have nonprofits that offer free or low-cost legal assistance for employment and disability-related issues.

Your Healthcare Team: Social workers or patient navigators at your treatment center can often help you understand your options and connect you with resources.

A Final Thought

Understanding your legal rights and workplace accommodations can empower you to navigate this journey with greater confidence. The laws and protections in place are designed to support your health, career, and well-being. By advocating for yourself and seeking the help you need, you can create a work-life balance that prioritizes your healing while preserving your professional identity. Remember, you are not alone—there are resources, professionals, and loved ones ready to stand by you every step of the way.

Part V: Advocacy and Awareness

Chapter 19

Testicular Cancer Myths and Facts

Testicular cancer is one of the most treatable forms of cancer, particularly when detected early. Despite its relatively high survival rates, the topic is often shrouded in myths and misconceptions that can lead to fear, stigma, or even delayed diagnosis. This chapter will address some of the most common myths surrounding testicular cancer, providing factual clarity and discussing related topics such as bilateral testicular cancer and genetic factors.

Common Misconceptions About Testicular Cancer

Myth 1: Testicular Cancer Only Affects Older Men Fact: Testicular cancer is most common in younger men, typically between the ages of 15 and 35. However, it can occur at any age, including in children and older adults. This misconception can lead to delayed diagnosis among younger men who don't consider themselves at risk. Regular self-examinations are crucial for early detection.

Myth 2: Testicular Cancer Is Always Fatal Fact: Testicular cancer has one of the highest survival rates among all cancers.

According to the American Cancer Society, the five-year survival rate for localized testicular cancer is over 95%. Even in advanced cases, treatments like chemotherapy and surgery are often highly effective. Early detection significantly improves outcomes.

Myth 3: Testicular Cancer Causes Immediate and Noticeable Symptoms Fact: In some cases, testicular cancer can be asymptomatic, especially in its early stages. When symptoms do occur, they may include a lump or swelling in the testicle, a feeling of heaviness in the scrotum, or dull pain in the lower abdomen or groin. Men should perform monthly self-exams and consult a healthcare provider if they notice any changes.

Myth 4: Only Men Can Develop Testicular Cancer Fact: While testicular cancer predominantly affects men, individuals assigned male at birth who later transition or identify differently can also develop this cancer. Understanding and addressing testicular cancer in diverse populations is vital for inclusive healthcare.

Myth 5: Injury to the Testicles Can Cause Cancer Fact: Injuries, such as being hit or struck in the testicles, do not cause cancer. However, they may prompt individuals to examine themselves, leading to the discovery of unrelated lumps or abnormalities. While a doctor should always check these, trauma is not a direct cause of cancer.

Myth 6: Fertility Is Always Lost After Testicular Cancer Fact: While some treatments for testicular cancer, such as chemotherapy or radiation, can impact fertility, this is not always the case. Many men retain their ability to father children after treatment. For those concerned about fertility, sperm banking before treatment is a recommended option.

Myth 7: Testicular Cancer Only Occurs in One Testicle Fact: While most cases involve one testicle, it is possible for testicular cancer to occur in both testicles, either simultaneously or at different times. This rare condition is known as bilateral testicular cancer and will be discussed in more detail below.

Clarifying Bilateral Testicular Cancer

Bilateral testicular cancer is uncommon, accounting for less than 5% of all testicular cancer cases. It can occur in two ways:

Synchronous Bilateral Testicular Cancer: Cancer develops in both testicles simultaneously. This is exceedingly rare.

Metachronous Bilateral Testicular Cancer: Cancer occurs in one testicle first and, after a period of remission, develops in the other testicle.

Key Considerations for Bilateral Testicular Cancer:

Diagnosis: Regular self-examinations and imaging techniques such as ultrasounds are critical for detecting abnormalities in both testicles.

Treatment: Treatment typically involves surgery (orchiectomy) and may include radiation or chemotherapy depending on the stage and spread of the cancer.

Hormonal Implications: Removing both testicles leads to a loss of testosterone production, requiring hormone replacement therapy to maintain overall health and quality of life.

Fertility Concerns: Fertility preservation options, such as sperm banking, are especially important for men facing bilateral cancer.

While bilateral testicular cancer poses additional challenges, advancements in medical care have greatly improved outcomes, allowing many patients to live full and healthy lives.

Genetic Factors and Testicular Cancer

Understanding the role of genetics in testicular cancer can provide insight into risk factors and prevention:

Family History: Men with a family history of testicular cancer, particularly a father or brother who has had the disease, are at higher risk. This doesn't mean they will definitely develop cancer, but it emphasizes the importance of regular monitoring.

Genetic Mutations: Certain genetic mutations, such as abnormalities in the KITLG gene, have been linked to increased susceptibility to testicular cancer. Research is ongoing to understand these genetic factors and their implications better.

Congenital Conditions: Some congenital conditions, such as undescended testicles (cryptorchidism), are associated with a higher risk of testicular cancer. Even if corrective surgery (orchiopexy) is performed, the risk remains elevated compared to the general population.

Environmental Interactions: Genetics may interact with environmental factors, such as exposure to certain chemicals or hormones, potentially increasing cancer risk. However, the exact mechanisms are not yet fully understood.

Genetic Counseling: Men with a strong family history or known genetic predisposition may benefit from genetic counseling. This involves discussing risk factors, testing options, and personalized recommendations for monitoring or preventive measures.

Debunking Fear Through Knowledge

Myths about testicular cancer can create unnecessary fear or lead to delayed medical care. By arming yourself with facts, you empower yourself or your loved ones to take proactive steps toward early detection and treatment. Here are a few steps to help overcome misinformation:

Educate Yourself: Use trusted resources such as the American Cancer Society, Mayo Clinic, or National Cancer Institute for accurate information.

Advocate for Regular Self-Exams: Encourage men to perform monthly self-checks, looking for changes in size, shape, or texture.

Spread Awareness: Use your voice to dispel myths within your community, creating a culture of openness and support around men's health.

Prioritize Medical Checkups: If something feels off, consult a doctor. Early diagnosis can make all the difference in successful treatment.

A Final Thought

Testicular cancer may be a daunting diagnosis, but it's also a disease with high survivability when addressed promptly. By debunking myths and highlighting facts, we can empower men to take control of their health. Whether it's through regular self-exams, seeking medical advice, or educating others, proactive measures save lives. Remember, knowledge is power—and with the right information, testicular cancer can be faced with confidence and resilience.

Benjamin's Story: A Journey of Strength, Support, and Gratitude

Benjamin Peterson's life took a sharp turn on February 9, 2024, when he was diagnosed with stage 3 choriocarcinoma that originated in his left testicle. The aggressive nature of his cancer was overwhelming, and the uncertainty was terrifying. "Choriocarcinoma" was a word that struck fear in his doctors, and it soon struck fear in him too. The initial shock of the diagnosis led to an immediate uprooting of his life—work was put on hold, future plans were paused, and his sole focus became getting to MD Anderson Hospital in Houston to begin treatment.

Benjamin underwent four cycles of BEP chemotherapy, a grueling regimen that tested his physical and emotional limits. Despite the challenges, he leaned heavily on the unwavering support of his wife, family, and friends. The love and encouragement he received—from surprise visits by loved ones to the compassion of the hospital staff—became the foundation of his fight.

The journey was far from easy. The fatigue, changes in taste, hair loss, and the emotional weight of facing his own mortality were constant battles. Even after treatment ended, the emotional toll lingered. Depression, anxiety, and the fear of recurrence became new obstacles to overcome. Through it all, Benjamin found solace in small joys—daily walks, time with loved ones, and moments of laughter that reminded him of the beauty in life.

Chapter 20

Engaging Young Men in Awareness

Talking about testicular cancer isn't exactly a locker room conversation, but it should be. The reality is, testicular cancer is the most common cancer in men aged 15 to 35. Yet, for many young men, it's barely on the radar. That's a problem we can fix by starting honest, straightforward conversations about testicular health. When young men are armed with knowledge, they're more likely to take action—whether that's performing self-exams, seeking medical advice, or supporting others who might be going through a diagnosis.

This chapter is about stepping up and changing the way we talk about men's health. It's about promoting support, breaking the stigma, and making sure guys know what to look for and how to act when it comes to testicular cancer.

Promoting Awareness in Communities

Awareness starts with education, but to reach young men effectively, you have to meet them where they are. Whether it's in schools, through sports teams, or on social media, the message needs to be clear: taking care of your health doesn't make you weak—it makes you smart.

1. Making the Message Relatable

One of the biggest barriers to awareness is the perception that talking about health is awkward or uncool. To overcome that, we need to make the message relatable and, dare we say, even a little bold. Humor, straightforward language, and real-life stories go a long way in grabbing attention.

Example: Campaigns like TCF's use phrases like "Check Your Balls" to make self-exams a normal part of the conversation. A little humor breaks the ice and gets guys talking.

Real Stories: Hearing from survivors who share their experiences in a no-nonsense way helps put a human face on the issue.

2. Starting the Conversation Early

Reaching young men in high school or college is crucial. Partnering with educational institutions and sports programs can help get the message out. Coaches, teachers, and mentors can all play a role in normalizing conversations about testicular health.

Workshops and Seminars: Offering short, engaging sessions on testicular cancer and self-exams can make a big impact.

Athlete Outreach: Tying awareness to athletic programs is especially effective. After all, athletes know their bodies better than most and understand the importance of maintaining good health.

Effective Communication About Testicular Health

Talking about testicular cancer doesn't have to be uncomfortable, but it does need to be clear and direct. Here's how to approach the conversation so it resonates with young men.

1. Keep It Simple

No one wants to sit through a lecture filled with medical jargon. Stick to the basics:

What is testicular cancer? A cancer that starts in the testicles, which is most common in young men.

What are the symptoms? A lump, swelling, or pain in the testicle. Simple, right?

What should you do? Perform monthly self-exams and see a doctor if something feels off.

2. Emphasize Early Detection

The earlier testicular cancer is caught, the better the outcomes. When young men know that performing a quick self-exam can save their lives, they're more likely to do it.

Practical Tips: Teach them how to do a self-exam. (Pro tip: it's easiest to do in the shower when the scrotum is relaxed.)

Positive Outcomes: Share that testicular cancer has a 95% survival rate when detected early. That's a statistic worth shouting about.

Breaking the Stigma

Let's face it: some guys might feel awkward talking about testicular health. That's where it's important to normalize these conversations and break down the stigma.

1. Build a Culture of Support

Create environments where men feel comfortable discussing their health. Whether it's a sports team, a fraternity, or a workplace, normalizing these conversations starts with leaders stepping up.

Survivor Stories: Hearing from other men who've been through testicular cancer can help break the ice.

Peer Advocacy: Encourage guys to remind their friends to perform self-exams or see a doctor if something seems wrong.

2. Get the Message Online

Young men spend a lot of time online, so digital campaigns are a powerful tool for raising awareness. Social media platforms are perfect for spreading messages that are short, bold, and to the point.

Hashtag Campaigns: Encourage young men to share messages like #CheckYourBalls to create a ripple effect of awareness.

Engaging Content: Use videos, memes, and infographics to make the topic approachable and shareable.

Creating Long-Term Change

Promoting awareness isn't just a one-time effort—it's about creating lasting change. Here's how to build a movement that sticks:

1. Empowering Young Men as Advocates

When guys take ownership of the issue, they become powerful advocates. Encourage young men to share what they've learned with their peers, creating a ripple effect of awareness.

Mentorship Programs: Pair survivors or older advocates with younger men to share their experiences and advice.

Ambassador Roles: Enlist young men to act as ambassadors for testicular health awareness in their schools, workplaces, or communities.

2. Partnering with Organizations Like TCF

The Testicular Cancer Foundation is at the forefront of spreading awareness and providing support. Partnering with organizations like TCF amplifies the message and provides resources for young men to take action.

Educational Materials: TCF provides guides and resources that make it easy to share the message.

Events and Campaigns: Join TCF events, such as their Annual Summit, or participate in their awareness campaigns to help make a bigger impact.

Final Thoughts on Engaging Young Men

Getting young men to care about testicular health isn't just about saving lives—it's about giving them the tools and confidence to take charge of their own health. When we talk openly, break the stigma, and make awareness relatable, we empower a generation to prioritize their well-being.

This isn't just a conversation; it's a movement. By spreading the word and supporting one another, we can ensure that testicular cancer is caught early, treated effectively, and—most importantly—that no one faces it alone. Let's step up, speak out, and make testicular health a priority. It's time to check in, take action, and keep the conversation going.

IF THESE BALLS COULD TALK

Chapter 21

Steps to Become an Advocate

Surviving testicular cancer or supporting someone through it is an experience that changes you. For many, it sparks a desire to give back and help others who may face the same battle. Advocacy is a powerful way to turn your experience into a force for good. By raising awareness, promoting early detection, and providing support to others, you can play a vital role in fighting testicular cancer.

This chapter is your roadmap to becoming an advocate. Whether you want to share your story, volunteer your time, or work with organizations like the Testicular Cancer Foundation (TCF), there's a way for you to get involved and make a meaningful impact.

Why Advocacy Matters

Advocacy isn't just about spreading awareness—it's about driving real change. By stepping into this role, you help educate others, save lives, and create a stronger community for those affected by testicular cancer.

1. Increasing Awareness

Many men don't think about testicular cancer until it affects them or someone they know. Advocates bring this conversation into the open, encouraging early detection and reducing the stigma around men's health.

2. Supporting Other Men

Sharing your story or simply being available to talk can provide invaluable comfort to those navigating their diagnosis. Advocacy fosters connections and reminds men they're not alone.

3. Contributing to a Bigger Cause

Your efforts help support research, improve resources, and push for better policies that benefit current and future patients.

Getting Started as an Advocate

You don't have to be a public speaker or medical expert to be an advocate. All it takes is a willingness to get involved and share your passion for making a difference. Here's how you can start:

1. Share Your Story

Your experience is powerful, and sharing it can inspire others to act. Whether you've been through treatment, supported a loved one, or simply want to help, your voice matters.

Social Media: Use platforms like Instagram, Facebook, or TikTok to share your journey. Authentic posts can reach a wide audience and make a lasting impact.

Community Events: Speak at schools, health fairs, or local organizations to promote awareness.

Online Forums: Join TCF's Discord community or other online spaces where you can connect with others and share your insights.

2. Get Educated

Before stepping into an advocacy role, it's important to understand the basics of testicular cancer. TCF offers educational resources that cover everything from early detection to treatment options.

Self-Exams: Learn how to perform and teach monthly self-exams. Advocates often focus on encouraging young men to check themselves regularly.

Statistics and Facts: Familiarize yourself with key information, like survival rates and common symptoms, to confidently answer questions and spread accurate knowledge.

3. Participate in Awareness Campaigns

Joining campaigns is a great way to amplify your voice and reach more people. TCF hosts several initiatives that make advocacy easy and impactful.

Annual Events: TCF's Annual Summit and regional meetups provide opportunities to connect with other advocates, share ideas, and build momentum.

Social Media Challenges: Get involved in TCF's online campaigns, like #CheckYourBalls, to encourage men to prioritize their health in a relatable way.

Partnering with Organizations Like TCF

The Testicular Cancer Foundation is a leader in awareness, education, and support for men affected by testicular cancer. Partnering with TCF gives you access to resources and a platform to make a bigger impact.

1. Volunteer with TCF

Volunteering is one of the easiest ways to get involved. Whether it's helping at events, mentoring newly diagnosed patients, or raising funds, your time and energy can make a difference.

2. Become a Mentor

TCF's mentorship programs connect survivors with those currently navigating their diagnosis. As a mentor, you provide guidance, answer questions, and offer encouragement based on your own experience.

3. Advocate Locally

TCF can support you in organizing local events or initiatives, like hosting a fundraiser, running a health seminar, or distributing educational materials in your community.

Steps to Take Your Advocacy to the Next Level

If you're ready to make a bigger impact, there are advanced ways to contribute to the fight against testicular cancer.

1. Fundraising for Research and Support

Raising money helps fund research, education programs, and resources for patients. TCF provides tools and support to help advocates run successful fundraisers.

Host Events: Organize a local 5K run, sports tournament, or charity auction to bring your community together for the cause.

Online Fundraising: Use platforms like GoFundMe or TCF's fundraising tools to reach a broader audience.

2. Advocate for Policy Changes

Advocacy at the policy level can drive systemic improvements in how testicular cancer is addressed.

Promote Awareness in Schools: Work with local schools to include information about testicular cancer in health classes.

Meet with Lawmakers: Advocate for better funding for testicular cancer research and awareness campaigns.

3. Build a Network

Strong advocacy relies on teamwork. Partner with other survivors, caregivers, and organizations to amplify your efforts.

The Impact of Advocacy

Advocates are the backbone of the testicular cancer community. Your efforts can lead to:

Early Detection: When more men know the signs and perform self-exams, more cases are caught early, leading to better outcomes.

Stronger Communities: Advocacy fosters connections, creating a network of support for patients and their families.

A Legacy of Awareness: By speaking out, you help normalize conversations about testicular cancer, breaking the stigma for future generations.

Final Thoughts on Becoming an Advocate

Stepping into advocacy is about more than just raising awareness—it's about using your experience to create change. Whether you're sharing your story, partnering with TCF, or organizing a community event, your efforts can save lives and make the journey easier for others.

Advocacy isn't a one-size-fits-all role. It's about finding what works for you and taking action. So, step up, speak out, and join the fight against testicular cancer. Your voice matters, and together, we can make a difference.

Sébastien's Story: From Nurse to Patient

Sébastien's battle with testicular cancer began unexpectedly in July 2010, just after the Football World Cup final. As a registered nurse from Basel, Switzerland, his life revolved around clinical work and cancer research, yet nothing could have prepared him for being on the receiving end of a life-altering diagnosis. What started as a dull heaviness in his right testicle soon became persistent pain and a noticeable nodule. After consulting a colleague and undergoing further examinations, the reality hit hard—testicular carcinoma.

That night in the hospital, the on-call urologist delivered the news with a mixture of urgency and reassurance. The cancer needed immediate surgical intervention, and within an hour, Sébastien was prepped for an orchiectomy. The whirlwind of emotions left him reeling—fear, uncertainty, and a desperate hope for a positive outcome. As a healthcare professional, he had seen countless patients face similar diagnoses, but experiencing it firsthand brought an entirely new level of vulnerability.

IF THESE BALLS COULD TALK

Chapter 22

Sharing Personal Stories

There's nothing tougher or more courageous than taking what you've been through and using it to help someone else. Testicular cancer is a life-altering experience, and the journey isn't always easy. But sharing your personal story—your raw, unfiltered truth—can be a lifeline for someone just starting their own fight.

Your story isn't just about you. It's a tool to educate, inspire, and create awareness. Whether you're helping another man feel less alone, encouraging someone to check themselves, or breaking down the stigma of talking about men's health, storytelling is a powerful way to make a difference.

Why Sharing Stories Matters

Your experience can resonate with others in a way no statistic or medical professional ever could. Here's why your story is important:

1. Building Awareness

When you share your journey, you're shining a light on a disease that many men don't think about until it's too late. By talking openly about your diagnosis, treatment, and recovery, you help others understand the importance of early detection and self-exams.

2. Offering Support

Hearing from someone who's been there can be a game-changer for someone navigating a diagnosis. Your story can provide comfort, hope, and practical advice during one of the scariest times in their life.

3. Breaking Stigma

Men's health issues are often swept under the rug. By speaking out, you're helping normalize conversations about testicular cancer, making it easier for other men to seek help and take action.

How to Share Your Story

You don't have to be a professional speaker or writer to share your experience. What matters most is authenticity—being real and honest about what you've been through.

1. Find Your Platform

Your story can reach people in different ways. Choose the platform that feels most comfortable and effective for you.

One-on-One Conversations: Talking directly with someone who's been diagnosed or is worried about their health can be deeply impactful.

Social Media: Platforms like Instagram, Facebook, or TikTok allow you to share your journey with a broad audience. Videos, photos, and posts can bring your story to life.

Support Groups: TCF's Discord community or weekly Zoom calls provide safe spaces to share your story with others who understand what you've been through.

Public Speaking: If you're comfortable, consider speaking at local events, health fairs, or TCF's Annual Summit. Sharing your journey face-to-face can inspire action and connection.

2. Be Honest and Vulnerable

The most powerful stories are the ones that show the real ups and downs. Don't be afraid to talk about the tough moments, but also highlight the lessons you've learned and the strength you've gained.

3. Focus on the Impact

When sharing your story, think about the message you want to convey. Maybe it's the importance of early detection, the value of support systems, or the need for better awareness campaigns. Your story can carry a message that motivates others to act.

The Ripple Effect of Storytelling

When you share your story, the impact doesn't stop with the person who hears it. Every man you inspire to perform a self-exam, every survivor you give hope to, and every caregiver you encourage to keep going becomes part of a chain reaction of awareness and support.

1. Inspiring Action

Your story can push someone to take that critical first step, whether it's seeing a doctor about a symptom, supporting a loved one through treatment, or joining a support group.

2. Spreading Awareness

Every conversation about testicular cancer helps normalize the topic and spreads the word about prevention and early detection.

3. Empowering Others to Share

When you open up, you give others the courage to do the same. One story inspires another, creating a community of voices that can't be ignored.

Sharing Stories Through TCF

The Testicular Cancer Foundation (TCF) provides platforms and opportunities for survivors to share their stories, amplifying their voices to make a bigger impact.

1. Join TCF's Support Network

TCF offers several ways to connect with others and share your journey, including their Discord community, weekly Zoom calls, and regional meetups. These are spaces where your story can encourage and inspire others in similar situations.

2. Participate in Events

TCF's Annual Summit and awareness campaigns provide opportunities to share your story with a larger audience. Whether you're speaking at an event or contributing to social media campaigns, your voice can make a difference.

3. Mentor Others

TCF's mentorship programs connect survivors with newly diagnosed patients. As a mentor, you can share your experience, answer questions, and provide the kind of understanding only someone who's been through it can offer.

Tips for Sharing Effectively

If you're ready to share your story, here are some tips to help you make the most impact:

Keep It Simple: Focus on the key moments and lessons from your journey. You don't need to include every detail.

Speak from the Heart: Authenticity is what resonates most with people. Don't worry about being perfect—just be yourself.

Be Positive but Realistic: Share hope and encouragement, but don't shy away from the challenges. Balance is key.

Engage Your Audience: Whether you're speaking in person or posting online, invite questions and interaction. The more engaged your audience, the greater the impact.

Final Thoughts on Sharing Stories

Your story has the power to change lives. It can educate, inspire, and create a ripple effect of awareness and action. Sharing your experience isn't just about looking back—it's about moving forward and using what you've learned to make a difference for others.

So, speak up. Whether it's in a one-on-one conversation, on social media, or at a TCF event, your voice matters. By sharing your story, you're not just contributing to the fight against testicular cancer—you're leading it. Let your experience be the spark that encourages men everywhere to take charge of their health and live stronger, more informed lives.

Conclusion Taking Action: The Fight Against Testicular Cancer Starts With You

As you've journeyed through this book, you've learned about the realities of testicular cancer, from recognizing early symptoms to navigating treatment, recovery, and advocacy. Whether you're a survivor, a caregiver, or someone passionate about raising awareness, you now have the tools to make a difference—not just in your own life but in the lives of countless others.

Let's take a moment to recap the key takeaways and focus on how you can step up, speak out, and help fight testicular cancer.

Summary of Key Takeaways

1. Awareness Saves Lives

Testicular cancer is one of the most treatable cancers, but early detection is critical. Regular self-exams, knowing the warning signs, and acting quickly can mean the difference between an easy recovery and a tougher fight. Every man should make it a habit to check himself monthly and talk to a doctor about any changes.

2. Support Systems Are Essential

No one should face testicular cancer alone. Whether it's a close friend, family member, or a community like the Testicular Cancer Foundation's network, having people to lean on is a game-changer. Support systems provide strength, understanding, and encouragement during one of the most challenging times in life.

3. Survivorship Is Just the Beginning

Life after treatment can bring its own challenges—physically, emotionally, and socially. Recovery takes time, but with the right resources, rehabilitation, and mindset, survivors can rebuild stronger lives. Sharing your story, mentoring others, and engaging in advocacy are powerful ways to turn your experience into a source of hope for others.

4. Advocacy Matters

Testicular cancer awareness needs champions. By talking openly about your journey, participating in events, or simply encouraging a friend to perform a self-exam, you're helping break the stigma and save lives.

Reinforcement of Awareness, Early Detection, and Support

Testicular cancer isn't just a medical issue—it's a community issue. The more men are aware of the risks and signs, the better equipped they are to take control of their health. Early detection leads to easier treatments and better outcomes, but it requires vigilance and education.

Support, whether from friends, family, or organizations like the Testicular Cancer Foundation, is the backbone of this fight. Knowing you're not alone makes the journey more manageable and provides the strength needed to keep moving forward.

Call to Action

Now it's your turn to take action. Whether you've been directly affected by testicular cancer or simply want to be part of the solution, there are ways for everyone to get involved.

1. Perform Regular Self-Exams

The first step is taking care of yourself. Make self-exams a routine part of your health check. If you notice anything unusual, don't wait—see a doctor.

2. Spread the Word

Talk to your friends, brothers, sons, and colleagues. Share what you've learned about testicular cancer and encourage them to prioritize their health. Join awareness campaigns, post on social media, and start conversations that matter.

3. Get Involved with TCF

The Testicular Cancer Foundation provides numerous opportunities to make a meaningful difference. Whether it's participating in their events, joining their online community, or becoming an advocate, your efforts can help save lives.

4. Support the Cause

Advocacy and research require resources. Consider donating to organizations like TCF or organizing fundraisers to support their mission. Every dollar helps educate more men, fund vital research, and provide resources for patients and survivors.

Final Words

Testicular cancer doesn't have to be faced in silence or shame. Every conversation you start, every self-exam you perform, every moment you choose awareness over ignorance—these are acts of courage that ripple outward, touching lives you may never see.

This isn't just about surviving a diagnosis. It's about transforming a culture that has taught men to suffer quietly, to ignore warning signs, to prioritize stoicism over survival. You now carry knowledge that can save lives—starting with your own.

Check yourself. Know your body. Trust your instincts when something feels wrong. And when you're ready, share what you've learned. Tell your son. Warn your brother. Be honest with your friends because the man whose life you save might be someone you love.

The statistics don't have to stay grim. The survival rates are already among the highest of any cancer, but only when caught early. That early detection depends on men like you breaking the silence.

Your voice matters. Your vigilance matters. Your willingness to have uncomfortable conversations matters.

The fight against testicular cancer doesn't start with researchers in labs or doctors in hospitals—it starts with men who refuse to look away. It starts with you.